HE
MEDICAL BOOK
OF LISTS

A PRIMER OF DIFFERENTIAL DIAGNOSIS IN INTERNAL MEDICINE

THE MEDICAL BOOK OF LISTS

A Primer of Differential Diagnosis
In Internal Medicine

FOURTH EDITION

NORTON J. GREENBERGER, MD,
*Peter T. Bohan Professor and Chairman,
Department of Medicine
University of Kansas Medical Center
Kansas City, Kansas*

SCOTT COONROD, MD,
*Former Chief Resident
Department of Medicine
University of Kansas Medical Center
Kansas City, Kansas*

CURTIS KAUER, MD,
*Former Chief Resident
Department of Medicine
University of Kansas Medical Center
Kansas City, Kansas*

MICHAEL LAWSON, MD,
*Former Chief Resident
Department of Medicine
University of Kansas Medical Center
Kansas City, Kansas*

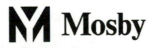

St. Louis   Baltimore   Berlin   Boston   Carlsbad   Chicago   London   Madrid
Naples   New York   Philadelphia   Sydney   Tokyo   Toronto

❚❱ Mosby

Acquisition Editor: Stephanie Manning
Managing Editor: Laura De Young
Project Manager: Barbara Bowes Merritt
Editing and Production: Page Two Associates, Inc.
Manufacturing Supervisor: Kathy Grone
Cover Design: Page Two Associates, Inc.

Fourth Edition
Copyright © 1994 by Mosby-Year Book, Inc.

Printed in the United States of America
Composition by Page Two Associates, Inc.
Printing/binding by Malloy

Mosby-Year Book, Inc.
11830 Westline Industrial Drive
St. Louis, Missouri 63146

Library of Congress Cataloging-in-Publication Data

The Medical Book of Lists: a primer of differential diagnosis/
     Norton Greenberger...[et al]. —4th ed.
        p.   cm.
     Includes bibliographical references.
     ISBN 0-8151-3437-1
     1. Diagnosis, Differential—Handbooks, manuals, etc.
I. Greenberger, Norton J.
     [DNLM: 1. Diagnosis, Differential—handbooks   WB 39M489]
RC71.5M38 1994
616.07'5—dc20   94-12103
DNLM/DLC   CIP
for Library of Congress

94 95 96 97 98 / 9 8 7 6 5 4 3 2 1

To my wife, Joan Narcus Greenberger, for her superb redactory efforts in reviewing all the tables in all four editions of this textbook.

PREFACE

The fourth edition of this book expands on the format of the first three editions, which have been well received by students, house officers, and faculty, and for which the authors are most appreciative.

Two of the most important considerations in the practice of internal medicine are the formulation of the differential diagnosis and the recognition of precise criteria on which to base a specific diagnosis. We have written this book because we believe that there is a need for a reasonably brief treatise that deals primarily with differential diagnosis. The book is a direct outgrowth of morning report sessions at the University of Kansas Medical Center. At these sessions, cases are presented as "unknowns" and resident physicians are asked to develop a differential diagnosis and also to indicate the specific criteria necessary to establish various diagnoses. This book, which contains over 250 lists, is a selective distillation of topics covered at morning report exercises. As such, the book is not a substitute for standard textbooks of medicine. Rather, it is viewed as a quick reference to key questions that may arise on ward rounds or at conference. The fourth edition has been extensively revised with several new tables and an entire chapter on AIDS.

Several individuals have made great contributions to this book. We thank several former chief residents and are especially indebted to our assistants Linda Taylor, Shirley Sears, and Ruth Stricklen for their preparation of the manuscript.

Norton J. Greenberger, MD
Scott Coonrod, MD
Curtis Kauer, MD
Michael Lawson, MD

CONTENTS

I. CARDIOLOGY

I-1	Innocent Murmurs	2
I-2	Causes of Splitting of the Second Heart Sound	2-3
I-3	Causes of Single Second Heart Sound	3
I-4	Physiological Classification of Continuous Murmurs	4
I-5	Mechanisms of Continuous Murmurs	4
I-6	Guidelines for the Diagnosis of Initial attack of Rheumatic Fever (Jones Criteria, 1992 Update)	5
I-7	Causes of Mitral Regurgitation	5-6
I-8	Etiology of Chronic and Acute Aortic Regurgitation	6
I-9	Causes of Tricuspid Regurgitation	7
I-10	Classification of Atrial Septal Defects	7
I-11	Causes of Atrial Flutter and Atrial Fibrillation	7
I-12	Complications of Mitral Stenosis	8
I-13	Risk Factors for Atherosclerotic Heart Disease	8
I-14	Purposes of ECG Exercise Tests	9
I-15	Myocardial Infarction: Clinical and Hemodynamic Subsets	10
I-16	Nonatherosclerotic Causes of Myocardial Infarction	11
I-17	Prognostic Determinants in Ischemic Heart Disease	12
I-18	Pseudoinfarction ECG Patterns	13
I-19	Causes of Sudden, Nontraumatic Death	14
I-20	Risk Factors for Anticoagulation	15
I-21	Etiologic Classification of Cardiomyopathies	16-17
I-22	Congestive Heart Failure: Precipitating Causes	17
I-23	Reversible Causes of Congestive Heart Failure	18
I-24	Potential Life-threatening Complications of Acute Myocardial Infarction	18

I-25	Types of Hypertension	19-20
I-26	Factors Indicating an Adverse Prognosis in Hypertension	20-21
I-27	Etiology of Syncope, Weakness, and Faintness	21-22
I-28	Classification of Pericarditis	23-24
I-29	Etiology of Chronic Constrictive Pericarditis	24
I-30	Clinical Features of Constrictive Pericarditis (137 cases)	25
I-31	Etiology of Pericardial Effusion	26
I-32	Common Etiologies of Cardiac Tamponade	27
I-33	Predisposing Factors to Chronic Pulmonary Hypertension and Cor Pulmonale	28
I-34	Pulmonary Valvular Insufficiency	29
I-35	Factors Predisposing to Thromboembolism	29
I-36	Digitalis Intoxication	30
I-37	Assessment of Cardiovascular Risk in Patients Being Considered for Surgery	31
I-38	Classification of Antiarrhythmic Drugs According to Their Mechanism of Action	32
I-39	Definite Indications for Implanted Pacemaker	33
I-40	Indications for Clinical Electrophysiological Studies — Endocardial Electrical Stimulation	34-35
I-41	NBG Pacemaker Code (1987)	36
I-42	Causes of Shock and Initiating Mechanisms	37-38
I-43	Contraindications of Thrombolytic Therapy	39
I-44	Bacterial Endocarditis Prophylaxis	40-41

II. ENDOCRINOLOGY — METABOLISM

II-1	Disorders Associated with Hypopituitarism	44-45
II-2	Differential Diagnosis of Hyperprolactinemia	45
II-3	Clinical Features of Acromegaly	46
II-4	Features Commonly Associated with the Primary Empty Sella Syndrome	46
II-5	Physiological Classification of Galactorrhea	47
II-6	Differential Diagnosis of the Syndrome of Inappropriate Antidiuresis (SIADH)	47-48
II-7	Causes of Hyperthyroidism	49
II-8	Clinical Features of Hyperthyroidism	49
II-9	Causes of Hypothyroidism	50
II-10	Clinical Features of Hypothyroidism	50
II-11	Circumstances Associated with Altered Concentration of TBG	51
II-12	Thyroid Tumor: Histological Classification of Epithelial Thyroid Tumors According to the World Health Organization	52-53

II-13	States Associated with Decreased Peripheral Conversion of T4 to T3	53
II-14	Adrenal Cortical Insufficiency	54
II-15	Clinical Features of Addison's Disease	55
II-16	Cushing's Syndrome	55
II-17	Clinical Features of Cushing's Syndrome	56
II-18	Syndrome of Primary Aldosteronism	57
II-19	Classification of Secondary Hyperaldosteronism	58-59
II-20	Causes of Hypomagnesemia and Magnesium Depletion	60
II-21	Classification of Diabetes Mellitus	61
II-22	Precipitating Factors in Diabetic Ketoacidosis	62
II-23	Major Causes of Fasting Hypoglycemia	63
II-24	Insulin Resistant States	64
II-25	A Classification of the Obesities	65-66
II-26	Hypercalcemic Conditions Arranged by Category in Descending Order of Approximate Frequency	66
II-27	Hypoparathyroidism	67
II-28	Nonhypoparathyroid Hypocalcemia Conditions	67-68
II-29	Classification of Osteomalacia and Rickets	68-69
II-30	Classification of Osteoporosis	70
II-31	Clinical Risk Factors for Calcium Stone Formation	71
II-32	Causes of Hirsutism in Females	71
II-33	Causes of Amenorrhea	72
II-34	Differential Diagnosis of Gynecomastia	73
II-35	Classification of Hyperlipidemias Based on Lipoprotein Concentrations	74
II-36	Relative Atherogenicity of Individual Lipoprotein Particles	74
II-37	Primary Versus Secondary Hyperlipidemias	75
II-38	Some Organic Causes of Erectile Impotence in Men	75-76
II-39	Hypophosphatemia	77
II-40	Complications of Corticosteroid Therapy	77-78
II-41	Some Causes of Hyperlactemia	79
II-42	Late Complications of Diabetes Mellitus	80

III. GASTROENTEROLOGY

III-1	Classification of Esophageal Motility Disorders	82
III-2	Achalasia	83
III-3	Conditions Associated with Hypergastrinemia and Diagnosis of Zollinger-Ellison Syndrome (ZES)	84
III-4	Differential Diagnosis of Refractory Duodenal Ulceration	85
III-5	Delayed Gastric Emptying	86-87
III-6	Diagnosis of Anorexia Nervosa	87
III-7	Classification of the Malabsorption Syndrome	88-89
III-8	Diagnosis of Celiac Sprue	90

III-9	Celiac Sprue - Failure to Respond to Gluten-free Diet	90
III-10	Conditions Associated with Bacterial Overgrowth	90
III-11	Diagnosis of "Bacterial Overgrowth" Syndrome	90
III-12	Clinical Features of Zinc Deficiency	91
III-13	Differential Diagnosis of Regional Enteritis	91
III-14	Features Differentiating Idiopathic Ulcerative Colitis from Granulomatous Colitis	92
III-15	Systemic Manifestations of Ulcerative Colitis (UC) and Regional Enteritis (RE)	93
III-16	Diagnosis of Irritable Bowel Syndrome	94
III-17	Classification, Diagnosis, and Management of Chronic Diarrheal Disorders	95-97
III-18	Risk Factors for Developing Colon Cancer	98
III-19	Diagnosis of Chronic Alcoholism	99
III-20	Spectrum of Alcoholic Liver Disease	100
III-21	Clinical and Histological Features of Alcoholic Hepatitis	100-101
III-22	Hepatitis A	101
III-23	Hepatitis C	102
III-24	Hepatitis B	103-105
III-25	Etiology and Diagnosis of Chronic Active Liver Disease	106
III-26	Primary Biliary Cirrhosis	107
III-27	Common Precipitating Causes of Hepatic Encephalopathy	108-109
III-28	Differential Diagnosis of Ascities	109-110
III-29	Conditions Causing or Contributing to Postoperative Jaundice	111
III-30	Differential Diagnosis of Jaundice due to Intrahepatic Cholestasis	112
III-31	Differential Diagnosis of Iron Storage Disease and Clinical Features of Idiopathic Hemochromatosis	113
III-32	Comparison of the Clinical, Radiologic, and Pathologic Characteristics of Focal Nodular Hyperplasia, and Liver Cell Adenoma	114-115
III-33	Clinical Features of Hepatoma	116
III-34	Diagnosis of Wilson's Disease	117
III-35	Principle Alterations of Hepatic Morphology Produced by Some Commonly Used Drugs and Chemicals	118
III-36	Causes of Pancreatic Exocrine Insufficiency	119
III-37	Causes of Acute Pancreatitis	119-120
III-38	Factors Adversely Influencing Survival in Acute Pancreatitis	121
III-39	Complications of Acute Pancreatitis	122-123

III-40	Complications of Chronic Pancreatitis	123
III-41	Diagnosis of Exocrine Pancreatic Insufficiency (EPI)	124
III-42	Postcholecystectomy Syndrome	124
III-43	Criteria for Assessing Severity of Malnutrition	125
III-44	Differential Diagnosis of Hypoalbuminemia	125
III-45	Granulomatous Liver Disease	126
III-46	Delta Agent	127
III-47	Primary Sclerosing Cholangitis	128
III-48	Predisposing Factors for Cholesterol and Pigment Gallstone Formation	129
III-49	Causes of Fulminant Hepatic Failure	130

IV. HEMATOLOGY — ONCOLOGY

IV-1	Differential Diagnosis of Normochromic-Normocytic Anemia	132
IV-2	Differential Diagnosis of Microcytic-Hypochromic Anemia	133
IV-3	Differential Diagnosis of Macrocytic Anemias	133-135
IV-4	Differential Diagnosis of Hemolytic Anemias	135-136
IV-5	Differential Diagnosis of Pancytopenia	137
IV-6	Differential Diagnosis of Aplastic Anemia	138
IV-7	Differential Diagnosis of Neutropenia	139
IV-8	Differential Diagnosis of Neutrophilia	140
IV-9	Differential Diagnosis of Eosinophilia	141
IV-10	Differential Diagnosis of Basophilia	142
IV-11	Disorders Associated with Monocytosis	143
IV-12	Differential Diagnosis of Abnormalities Found on Peripheral Smear	143-144
IV-13	Differential Diagnosis of Erythrocytosis	145
IV-14	Criteria for the Diagnosis of Polycythemia Vera	146
IV-15	Differential Diagnosis of Thrombocytosis	147
IV-16	Myelodysplastic Syndromes	147
IV-17	Myeloproliferative Syndromes	147
IV-18	Staging of Chronic Lymphocytic Leukemia	148
IV-19	Criteria for the Diagnosis of Multiple Myeloma	148
IV-20	Staging System for Multiple Myeloma	149
IV-21	Renal and Electrolyte Disorders in Multiple Myeloma	150
IV-22	Criteria for the Diagnosis of Thrombotic Thrombocytopenic Purpura	150
IV-23	Differential Diagnosis of Splenomegaly	151
IV-24	Differential Diagnosis of Lymphadenopathy	152-153
IV-25	Differential Diagnosis of Thrombocytopenia	153
IV-26	Causes of Cyanosis	154
IV-27	Paraneoplastic Syndromes	155
IV-28	Causes of Hyponatremia in Cancer Patients	156

IV-29	Factors Related to the Survival of Patients with Breast Cancer	156
IV-30	TNM Nomenclature of Lung Cancers	157
IV-31	Stages of Lung Cancer According to TNM Nomenclature	157
IV-32	Most Frequent Types of Neoplasms in Malignant Pleural Effusions	158
IV-33	Most Frequent Malignancies Causing Peritoneal Effusions	158
IV-34	Most Frequent Neoplasms Causing Malignant Pericardial Effusion	158
IV-35	Etiological Factors of Hypercalcemia of Malignancy	159
IV-36	Cancers Most Likely to Metastasize to Bone	159
IV-37	General Responses of Various Malignancies to Antineoplastic Chemotherapy	160-161
IV-38	Long-Term Effects of Radiation	161
IV-39	Clinical Features of Graft-Versus-Host Disease	162
IV-40	Superior Vena Cava Syndrome	163
IV-41	Cauda Equina Syndrome	163
IV-42	Signs and Symptoms of Epidural Compression	163
IV-43	Cotswold Staging Classification of Hodgkins Disease	164
IV-44	Working Formulation of Non-Hodgkin's Lymphomas	165-166
IV-45	Performance Status Criteria (Karnofsky Scale)	167
IV-46	Multiple Endocrine Neoplasia Syndrome	168
IV-47	Risk Factors Predisposing to Thrombosis	169

V.   INFECTIOUS DISEASE

V-1	Disease States Causing Fever of Unknown Origin	172-173
V-2	Classification of Tuberculosis	173
V-3	Clinical Features of Genitourinary Tuberculosis	173
V-4	Criteria for the Diagnosis of Nontuberculosis Mycobacterial Disease in Nonimmunocompromised Hosts	174
V-5	Immunocompromised Hosts	174
V-6	Pulmonary Infections in Immunocompromised Patients	175
V-7	Clinical Pulmonary Syndromes of Histoplasmosis	175
V-8	Extrapulmonary Manifestations of Mycoplasma Pneumoniae	176
V-9	Extrapulmonary Manifestations of Psittacosis	177
V-10	Extrapulmonary Manifestations of Q Fever	177
V-11	Features of Legionella Infection	178
V-12	Clinical and Laboratory Features of Cytomegalovirus Mononucleosis (Non-immune Compromised Host)	179

V-13	Factors Associated with Mortality in Brain Abscess	180
V-14	Risk Factors Affecting Outcome of Bacteremia	181
V-15	Major Types of Osteomyelitis*	182-183
V-16	Spectrum of Gonococcal Infections	184
V-17	Clinical Features of Food Poisoning Secondary to Botulism	185
V-18	Antibiotic-Associated Pseudomembranous Colitis	186
V-19	Toxic Shock Syndrome	187
V-20	Anaerobic Infections	188
V-21	Listeria Monocytogenes Infections	189
V-22	Effective Drug Regimens for the Treatment of Tuberculosis	190-191
V-23	Manifestations of Lyme Disease by Stage	192-193
V-24	Chronic Fatigue Syndrome: Diagnostic Criteria	194-195

VI. NEPHROLOGY

VI-1	Differential Diagnosis of Metabolic Alkalosis	198
VI-2	Differential Diagnosis of Metabolic Acidosis with Increased Anion Gap	199
VI-3	Differential Diagnosis of Metabolic Acidosis with Normal Anion Gap (Hyperchloremic Acidosis)	200
VI-4	Differential Diagnosis of a Low Anion Gap	200
VI-5	Differential Diagnosis of Hypokalemia	201
VI-6	Differential Diagnosis of Hyperkalemia	202
VI-7	Differential Diagnosis of Hypernatremia	203
VI-8	Differential Diagnosis of Hyponatremia	204
VI-9	Differential Diagnosis of Renal Tubular Acidosis (RTA) Type I (Distal)	204-205
VI-10	Differential Diagnosis of Renal Tubular Acidosis (RTA) Type II (Proximal)	206
VI-11	Differential Diagnosis of Renal Tubular Acidosis (RTA) Type IV	207
VI-12	Differential Diagnosis of Parenchymal Renal Diseases Causing Acute Renal Failure	208
VI-13	Differential Diagnosis of Acute Deterioration in Renal Function	208-209
VI-14	Differential Diagnosis of Common Mechanical Causes of Urinary Tract Obstruction	210-211
VI-15	Major Nephrotoxins	212
VI-16	Differentiation of Dehydration and Acute Tubular Injury as a Cause of Oliguria	213
VI-17	Differential Diagnosis of Acute Glomerulonephritis	214
VI-18	Differential Diagnosis of the Nephrotic Syndrome	214-216
VI-19	Differential Diagnosis of Tubulointerstitial Disease of the Kidney	216-217

VI-20	Differential Diagnosis of Nephrogenic Diabetes Insipidus	217-218
VI-21	Differential Diagnosis of Central Diabetes Insipidus	218-219
VI-22	Differential Diagnosis of Hyperuricemia	219
VI-23	Differential Diagnosis of Nephrolithiasis	220
VI-24	Differential Diagnosis of Hypouricemia	220-221
VI-25	Renal Complications of Neoplasms	222
VI-26	Conditions Leading to Generalized Edema	223
VI-27	Clinical Spectrum of Abnormalities in Uremia	224-225
VI-28	Differential Diagnosis of Respiratory Acidosis	226
VI-29	Differential Diagnosis of Respiratory Alkalosis	227
VI-30	Rules of Thumb for Bedside Interpretation of Acid-Base Disorders	228
VI-31	Complications of Dialysis	229
VI-32	Causes of Hematuria	230-231

VII. PULMONARY DISEASE

VII-1	Differential Diagnosis of Clubbing of the Digits	234
VII-2	Differential Diagnosis of Hemoptysis	235
VII-3	Differential Diagnosis of Bronchiectasis	236
VII-4	Differential Diagnosis of Pleural Effusions	237
VII-5	Evaluation of Pleural Effusions	238
VII-6	Differential Diagnosis of Cough with Negative Chest X-Ray	239
VII-7	Differential Diagnosis of Hilar Enlargement	240
VII-8	Differential Diagnosis of Pneumothorax	241
VII-9	Differential Diagnosis of Recurrent Pulmonary Infection Associated with Immunodeficiency Syndromes other than HIV-Related	242
VII-10	Differential Diagnosis of Eosinophilic Lung Disease	243
VII-11	Differential Diagnosis of Pulmonary Interstitial Disease of Known Etiology	244
VII-12	Differential Diagnosis of Pulmonary Interstitial Disease of Unknown Etiology	244
VII-13	Differential Diagnosis of Respiratory Failure	245
VII-14	Guidelines for Withdrawal of Mechanical Ventilation	246
VII-15	Differential Diagnosis of Alveolar Hyperventilation	247
VII-16	Differential Diagnosis of Chronic Alveolar Hypoventilation	248
VII-17	Symptoms and Signs Observed in 327 Patients with Angiographically Documented Pulmonary Emboli	249
VII-18	ECG Changes in Pulmonary Embolism	250
VII-19	Clinical Disorders Associated with the Adult Respiratory Distress Syndrome	251
VII-20	Prognostic Indicators in Pneumococcal Pneumonia	252
VII-21	Classification of Lung Abscesses According to Cause	252

VII-22	Criteria for the Diagnosis of Allergic Bronchopulmonary Aspergillosis	253
VII-23	Solitary Pulmonary Nodules	254
VII-24	Differential Diagnosis of Tumors Metastatic to the Lungs	255
VII-25	Differential Diagnosis of a Mediastinal Mass	256-257
VII-26	Pulmonary Manifestations of the Collagen-Vascular Diseases	258
VII-27	Pulmonary-Renal Syndromes	259
VII-28	Imitators of Pulmonary-Renal Syndromes	259
VII-29	Differential Diagnosis of Fever and Pulmonary Infiltrates in Renal Transplants	260
VII-30	Drugs Implicated in the Etiology of Pulmonary Parenchymal Injury	261
VII-31	Multi-Organ System Failure: Modified Apache II Criteria	262

VIII. CLINICAL IMMUNOLOGY AND RHEUMATOLOGY

VIII-1	Diagnostic Criteria for Systemic Lupus Erythematosus	264
VIII-2	Underlying Conditions Associated with Raynaud's Phenomenon	265
VIII-3	Polymyalgia Rheumatica	266
VIII-4	Criteria for Diagnosis of Stevens-Johnson Syndrome	266
VIII-5	Diagnosis of Behçet's Syndrome	267
VIII-6	Criteria for the Diagnosis of Scleroderma (Progressive Systemic Sclerosis)	267
VIII-7	Diagnosis Criteria for Inflammatory Myopathies	268-269
VIII-8	Revised Criteria for Classification of Rheumatoid Arthritis (Traditional Format)	270
VIII-9	Clinical Features Suggesting Reiter's Syndrome	271
VIII-10	Diagnostic Criteria of Ankylosing Spondylitis	271
VIII-11	Criteria for Diagnosis of Gouty Arthritis	272
VIII-12	Provisional Criteria for Diagnosis of Psoriatic Arthritis	272-273
VIII-13	Differential Diagnosis of Inflammatory Monoarthritis	273
VIII-14	Diagnostic Features of Sarcoidosis	274
VIII-15	Differential Diagnosis of Positive Blood Test for Rheumatoid Factor	275
VIII-16	Cryoglobulinemia	276
VIII-17	Classification of the Vasculitic Syndromes	277
VIII-18	Autoantibodies in Rheumatic Diseases: Disease Associations and Molecular Identification	278
VIII-19	Putative Associations of CPPD Crystal Deposition	279
VIII-20	Synovial Fluid Characteristics	280-281
VIII-21	The American College of Rheumatology 1990 Criteria for the Classification of Fibromyalgia	282

XVIII

IX. NEUROLOGY

IX-1	Classification of Coma and Differential Diagnosis	284
IX-2	Differential Diagnosis of Meningitis	285
IX-3	Differential Diagnosis of Peripheral Neuropathies	286
IX-4	Classification of Dementia	286-287
IX-5	Classification of Delirium and Acute Confusional States	287-288
IX-6	Secondary Causes of Depression	289
IX-7	Causes of Hypoglycorrhachia (Decreased Cerebrospinal Fluid Glucose)	290

X. DERMATOLOGY

X-1	Conditions Associated with Erythema Nodosum	292-293
X-2	Causes of Anhidrosis	293
X-3	Suspected Etiologic Factors in Erythema Multiforme	294
X-4	Clinical Manifestations of Mastocytosis	294
X-5	Classification of Cutaneous Signs of Internal Malignancy	295-296
X-6	Drugs that Cause Pruritus	297

XI. ACQUIRED IMMUNODEFICIENCY SYNDROME (AIDS)

XI-1	Diagnostic Criteria for Acquired Immunodeficiency Syndrome (AIDS)	300-301
XI-2	Relation of Clinical Manifestations to CD4 Count in HIV-Infected Patients	302
XI-3	Renal Syndromes in Patients with HIV Infection	303-304
XI-4	Major Endocrine Complications in Acquired Immunodeficiency Syndrome	305
XI-5	Gastrointestinal Manifestations of AIDS	306
XI-6	Gastrointestinal Pathogens in HIV-Infected Patients	307
XI-7	Rheumatologic Manifestations of Infection with Human Immunodeficiency Virus (HIV)	308
XI-8	AIDS Associated Hematologic Disorders	309
XI-9	Mucocutaneous Manifestations in AIDS	310
XI-10	Pulmonary Complications of HIV Infection	311
XI-11	Neurologic Problems in AIDS Patients	312
XI-12	Cancers in the HIV Epidemic	313

INDEX	315

THE
MEDICAL BOOK
OF LISTS

A PRIMER OF DIFFERENTIAL DIAGNOSIS
IN INTERNAL MEDICINE

CHAPTER I
CARDIOLOGY

I-1 INNOCENT MURMURS

I. Patients in whom innocent murmurs are more likely to occur
   A. Children and adolescents
   B. Pregnant women
   C. Anxious persons
   D. Funnel-breasted or flat-chested persons
   E. Persons with the straight-back syndrome
   F. Hyperthyroid and anemic persons

II. Types of innocent murmurs
Innocent murmurs may be classified as follows:
   A. Completely innocent
      1. Cervical venous hum
      2. Supraclavicular arterial bruit
      3. Still's murmur
      4. Mammary souffle
      5. Ejection systolic murmur in the pulmonary area
      6. Innocent abdominal murmurs
   B. Relatively innocent
      1. Early systolic murmur
      2. Pulmonary systolic murmur with high output states
         (hemic murmur)

I-2 CAUSES OF SPLITTING OF THE SECOND HEART SOUND

I. Delayed pulmonic closure
   Delayed electrical activation of the right ventricle
   A. Complete RBBB (proximal type)
   B. Left ventricular paced beats
   C. Left ventricular ectopic beats

II. Prolonged right ventricular mechanical systole
   A. Acute massive pulmonary embolus
   B. Pulmonary hypertension with right heart failure
   C. Pulmonic stenosis with intact septum (moderate to severe)

III. Decreased impedance of the pulmonary vascular bed
     (increased hang-out)
   A. Normotensive atrial septal defect
   B. Idiopathic dilatation of the pulmonary artery
   C. Pulmonic stenosis (mild)
   D. Atrial septal defect, postoperative (70%)

IV. Early aortic closure
   Shortened left ventricular mechanical systole (LVET)
   A. Mitral regurgitation
   B. Ventricular septal defect

I-2 CAUSES OF SPLITTING OF THE SECOND HEART SOUND (CONTINUED) REVERSED SPLITTING

  V. Delayed aortic closure
Delayed electrical activation of the left ventricle
- A. Complete LBBB (proximal type)
- B. Right ventricular paced beats
- C. Right ventricular ectopic beats

  VI. Prolonged left ventricular mechanical systole
- A. Complete LBBB (peripheral type)
- B. Left ventricular outflow tract obstruction
- C. Hypertensive cardiovascular disease
- D. Arteriosclerotic heart disease
  1. Chronic ischemic heart disease
  2. Angina pectoris

  VII. Decreased impedance of the systemic vascular bed (increased hang-out)
- A. Poststenotic dilatation of the aorta secondary to aortic stenosis or insufficiency
- B. Patent ductus arteriosus

  VIII. Early pulmonic closure
Early electrical activation of the right ventricle
- A. Wolff-Parkinson-White syndrome, type B

RBBB = right bundle-branch block; AES = audible expiratory splitting; LVET = left ventricular ejection time; LBBB = left bundle-branch block.

Reference: Perloff JK. In Braunwald E, et al, editors: *Heart disease: a textbook of cardiovascular medicine,* ed 4. Philadelphia,1992, W. B. Saunders, pp. 46-48.

I-3 CAUSES OF SINGLE SECOND HEART SOUND

    I. Tetralogy of Fallot
   II. Truncus and pseudotruncus arteriosus
  III. Very severe pulmonary valvular stenosis (occasional case)
  IV. Tricuspid atresia
   V. Aortic stenosis (occasional case)
  VI. Left bundle branch block (occasional case)
 VII. Age over 45 years (variable)
VIII. Eisenmenger's VSD
  IX. Severe semilunar valve disease
   X. Any of the causes of reversed splitting of second heart sound
  XI. One of the sounds inaudible (example, emphysema or obesity)

I-4 PHYSIOLOGIC CLASSIFICATION OF CONTINUOUS MURMURS

I. Continuous murmurs due to rapid blood flow
   A. Venous hum
   B. Mammary souffle
   C. Hemangioma
   D. Hyperthyroidism
   E. Acute alcoholic hepatitis
   F. Hyperemia of neoplasm (hepatoma, renal cell carcinoma, Paget's disease)

II. Continuous murmurs due to high-to-low pressure shunts
   A. Systemic artery to pulmonary artery (patent ductus arteriosus, aortopulmonary window, truncus arteriosus, pulmonary atresia, anomalous left coronary, bronchiectasis, sequestration of the lung)
   B. Systemic artery to right heart (ruptured sinus of Valsalva, coronary artery fistula)
   C. Left-to-right atrial shunting (Lutembacher's syndrome, mitral atresia plus atrial septal defect)
   D. Venovenous shunts (anomalous pulmonary veins, portosystemic shunts)
   E. A-V fistula (systemic or pulmonic)

III. Continuous murmurs secondary to localized arterial obstruction
   A. Coarctation of the aorta
   B. Branch pulmonary stenosis
   C. Carotid occlusion
   D. Celiac mesenteric occlusion
   E. Renal occlusion
   F. Femoral occlusion
   G. Coronary occlusion

From: Myers JD. The mechanisms and significances of continuous murmurs. In Leon DF, Shaver JA, editors, *Physiologic principles of heart sounds and murmurs*. New York, 1975, American Heart Association, Monograph 46, p. 202. As printed In: Hurst JW, et al, editors, *The heart*, ed 7. New York, 1990, McGraw-Hill, p. 232. Reproduced with permission from the American Heart Association, Inc. and the author.

I-5 MECHANISMS OF CONTINUOUS MURMURS

I. Connections between aorta and pulmonary artery
II. Arteriovenous fistulas
III. Turbulent flow in arteries
IV. Turbulent flow in veins
V. Communication between left and right atrium
VI. Rapid blood flow

I-6 GUIDELINES FOR THE DIAGNOSIS OF INITIAL ATTACK OF RHEUMATIC FEVER (JONES CRITERIA, 1992 UPDATE)

I. Major manifestations
   A. Carditis
   B. Polyarthritis
   C. Chorea
   D. Erythema marginatum
   E. Subcutaneous nodules
II. Minor manifestations
   A. Clinical findings
      1. Arthralgia
      2. Fever
   B. Laboratory findings
      1. Elevated acute phase reactants
      2. Erythrocyte sedimentation rate
      3. C-reactive protein
      4. Prolonged PR interval
III. Supporting evidence of antecedent group A streptococcal infection*
   A. Positive throat culture or rapid streptococcal antigen test
   B. Elevated or rising streptococcal antibody titer

*If supported by evidence of preceding group A streptococcal infection, the presence of two major manifestations or of one major and two minor manifestations indicates a high probability of acute rheumatic fever.

Adapted from: Special Writing Group. *JAMA* 268(15):2070, 1992.

I-7 CAUSES OF MITRAL REGURGITATION

I. Spontaneous rupture of chordae tendineae
II. Trauma
III. Mitral valve prolapse
IV. Ischemia
V. Myocardial infarction
VI. Aneurysm of left ventricle involving the mitral annulus
VII. Infective endocarditis
VIII. Congestive cardiomyopathies
IX. IHSS
X. Rheumatic heart disease
XI. SLE
XII. Scleroderma
XIII. Takayasu's arteritis
XIV. Myxomatous degeneration of mitral valve leaflets
XV. Calcified mitral annulus
XVI. Marfan's syndrome

I-7 CAUSES OF MITRAL REGURGITATION (CONTINUED)

XVII. Ehlers-Danlos syndrome
XVIII. Pseudoxanthoma elasticum
XIX. Ankylosing spondylitis
XX. Rheumatoid arthritis
XXI. Congenital (mitral valve clefts, endocardial cushion defects, endocardial fibroelastosis, transposition of the great arteries, anomalous origin of left coronary artery)

I-8 ETIOLOGY OF CHRONIC AND ACUTE AORTIC REGURGITATION

I. Chronic aortic regurgitation
   A. Rheumatic
   B. Syphilis
   C. Arteritis (Takayasu's)
   D. Aorticoannuloectasia
   E. Heritable disorders of connective tissue
      1. Marfan's syndrome
      2. Ehlers-Danlos syndrome
      3. Osteogenesis imperfecta
   F. Congenital heart disease
      1. Bicuspid aortic valve
      2. Interventricular septal defect
      3. Sinus of Valsalva aneurysm
   G. Arthritic diseases
      1. Ankylosing spondylitis
      2. Reiter's syndrome
      3. Rheumatoid arthritis
      4. Systemic lupus erythematosus
   H. Cystic medial necrosis of aorta
   I. Hypertension
   J. Arteriosclerosis
   K. Myxomatous degeneration of valve
   L. Infective endocarditis
   M. Following prosthetic valve surgery
   N. Associated with aortic stenosis
II. Acute aortic regurgitation
   A. Rheumatic fever
   B. Infective endocarditis
   C. Congenital (rupture of sinus of Valsalva)
   D. Acute aortic dissection
   E. Following prosthetic valve surgery
   F. Trauma

Please note that certain disorders are capable of producing acute and chronic aortic regurgitation.

From: Hurst JW, Rackley CE, Sonnenblick EH, Wenger NK, editors: *The heart*, ed 7. New York, 1990, McGraw-Hill, p. 806.

I-9 CAUSES OF TRICUSPID REGURGITATION

I. Rheumatic heart disease
II. Endocarditis
III. Myocardial infarction (with or without papillary muscle dysfunction)
IV. Trauma
V. Pulmonary hypertension
VI. Ebstein's anomaly
VII. Endocardial pacemaker wire
VIII. Pulmonary artery catheter (Swan-Ganz)
IX. Carcinoid
X. Rheumatoid arthritis
XI. Radiation
XII. Floppy (prolapse)

I-10 CLASSIFICATION OF ATRIAL SEPTAL DEFECTS

I. Patent foramen ovale
II. Persistent ostium secundum defect (fossa ovalis defect)
III. Sinus venosus defect (proximal defect)
IV. Endocardial cushion defect (complete and partial atrioventricular canal)
   A. Ostium primum defect (incomplete persistent common atrioventricular canal)
   B. Complete persistent common atrioventricular canal

I-11 CAUSES OF ATRIAL FLUTTER AND ATRIAL FIBRILLATION

I. Valvular heart disease (mitral or tricuspid stenosis or regurgitation)
II. Ischemic heart disease
III. Hypertensive heart disease
IV. Cardiomyopathy (dilated or hypertrophic)
V. Congenital heart disease (atrial septal defect)
VI. Pericarditis
VII. Mitral valve prolapse
VIII. Sick sinus syndrome
IX. Pulmonary embolism
X. Thyrotoxicosis
XI. Hypoxemia of any etiology
XII. Alcohol ingestion ("holiday heart syndrome")
XIII. Atrial infarction

Modified from: Walsh K, Ezri M, and Denes P. *Med Clin N Amer*, 70(4):794, 1986.

I-12 COMPLICATIONS OF MITRAL STENOSIS

I. Unrelated to severity of stenosis
   A. Atrial fibrillation
   B. Infective endocarditis
   C. Embolism
II. Related to severity of stenosis
   A. Pulmonary edema
   B. Hemoptysis
   C. Dyspnea on exertion
   D. Pulmonary hypertension
   E. Right ventricular failure
III. Chest x-ray findings in mitral stenosis
   A. Enlargement of left atrium
   B. Enlargement of right ventricle
   C. Kerley B lines
   D. Enlargement of the pulmonary artery
   E. Cephalization of the pulmonary vasculature
   F. Calcification in the area of the mitral valve

I-13 RISK FACTORS FOR ATHEROSCLEROTIC HEART DISEASE

I. Hypercholesterolemia — low HDL cholesterol
II. Hypertension
III. Tobacco use
IV. Diabetes mellitus (abnormal glucose tolerance)
V. Family history of atherosclerosis (M.I., stroke, peripheral vascular disease)
VI. Obesity
VII. Sedentary living
VIII. Type A personality
IX. Oral contraceptive use
X. Chronic obstructive lung disease
XI. Chronic renal failure
XII. Hypertriglyceridemia (Type IV)
XIII. Alcohol (greater than 3 oz. distilled liquor or equivalent)
XIV. Male (or postmenopausal female)
XV. Immunosuppressive posttransplant
XVI. Elevated fibrinogen
XVII. Syndrome X (hypertriglyceridemia, hypertension, insulin resistance, centripetal obesity).

Modified from: Farmer JA, Gotto AM. In Braunwald E, et al, editors: *Heart disease, a textbook of cardiovascular medicine*, ed 4. Philadelphia, 1992, W. B. Saunders, pp. 1125-1155.

I-14 PURPOSES OF ECG EXERCISE TESTS

I. Screening an asymptomatic population
   A. For prognostic evaluation, e.g., in general epidemiology surveys or of insurance applicants.
   B. For investigations of groups at high risk for coronary disease, e.g., hyperlipidemic patients.
   C. For study of workers in critical positions, e.g., commercial aircraft pilots, military pilots.
II. For diagnostic evaluation of patients with chest pain not typical of angina pectoris.
III. For evaluating the degree of ischemia in patients with known angina or previous infarction—with regard to prognosis, treatment, permitted exercise level.
IV. For evaluating therapeutic procedures in patients with angina, e.g., coronary artery bypass grafting or trial of new drugs.
V. For evaluating severity of other lesions, e.g., aortic stenosis in children, mitral stenosis (there is a general reluctance to exercise adults with aortic stenosis for fear of provoking ventricular arrhythmias).
VI. For evaluating work capacity, e.g., following cardiac infarction.
VII. To evaluate entry into or the results of rehabilitation or exercise training programs.
VIII. To evaluate patients suspected of AV block or sinus node dysfunction.

I-15 MYOCARDIAL INFARCTION: CLINICAL AND HEMODYNAMIC SUBSETS

I. Class I
  A. Clinical: No evidence of heart failure
  B. Hemodynamic: PCWP = NML; CI > 2.2
  C. Prognosis: In-hospital mortality 5% to 7%*

II. Class II
  A. Clinical: Tachycardia, bibasilar rales to scapula tip and/or S_3 gallop
  B. Hemodynamic: PCWP > 18 mm Hg; CI > 2.2
  C. Prognosis: In-hospital mortality 10% to 15%*

III. Class III
  A. Clinical: Tachycardia, rales above tip of scapula, S_3 gallop or frank pulmonary edema
  B. Hemodynamic: PCWP $\leq$ 18; CI < 2.2
  C. Prognosis: In hospital mortality 25% to 50%*

IV. Class IV (cardiogenic shock)
  A. Clinical: Hypotension, cool clammy extremities, mental confusion, decreased urine output
  B. Hemodynamic: PCWP > 18; CI < 2.2
  C. Prognosis: In-hospital mortality 80% to 90%*

*Current mortality may be lower (i.e., thrombolytics and angioplasty)
PCWP = Pulmonary capillary wedge pressure (mm Hg)
CI = Cardiac index (L/min/M²)

References: Killip T, III, and Kimball JT. Treatment of myocardial infarction in a coronary care unit. *Am J Cardiol* 20:457, 1967.
Forrester J, Waters D. Hospital treatment of congestive heart failure: management according to hemodynamic profile. *Am J Med* 65:73, 1978.

I-16 NONATHEROSCLEROTIC CAUSES OF MYOCARDIAL INFARCTION

I. Emboli to coronary arteries
   A. Thrombi from left ventricle (AMI, cardiomyopathy)
   B. Thrombi from left atrium (mitral stenosis)
   C. Thrombi from prosthetic valves
   D. Thrombi from catheters during angiography
   E. Air emboli (coronary angiography, cardiopulmonary bypass)
   F. Infectious and marantic endocarditis
   G. Atrial myxoma

II. Mechanical obstruction
   A. Chest trauma (contusion, laceration)
   B. Dissection of the aorta
   C. Dissection of coronary arteries (postpartum, post-PTCA, post-coronary angiography)

III. Increased vasomotor tone
   A. Variant angina
   B. Raynaud's disease
   C. Nitroglycerin withdrawal

IV. Arteritis
   A. Collagen vascular disease (PAN, SLE, RA, AS)
   B. Takayasu's disease
   C. Mucocutaneous lymph node (Kawasaki's) syndrome
   D. Luetic aortitis

V. Miscellaneous
   A. Anomalous origin and/or course of coronary arteries
   B. Hematologic disorders (DIC, PV)
   C. Aortic stenosis
   D. Hypertrophic cardiomyopathy
   E. Prolonged hypotension
   F. Cocaine

AMI = Anterior myocardial infarction
PTCA = Percutaneous transcoronary angioplasty
PAN = Polyarteritis nodosa
AS = Ankylosing spondylitis
PV = Polycythemia vera

Modified from: Cheitlin M, McAllister HA, Castro CM. Myocardial infarction without atherosclerosis. *JAMA* 231:951-955, 1975. Codini MA. *Med Clin N Amer* 70(4):771, 1986.

I-17 PROGNOSTIC DETERMINANTS IN ISCHEMIC HEART DISEASE

I. Objective severity of ischemia
   A. Treadmill
      1. Duration of exercise (failure to achieve 3 METS)
      2. Degree of ST depression/elevation during/post exercise
      3. Abnormal blood pressure response to exercise
      4. Exercise-induced ventricular ectopy
      5. Reversible ischemia with exercise by isotope
   B. Inability to perform exercise testing
II. Degree of left ventricular dysfunction
III. Recurrent ischemic events
   A. Myocardial infarction
   B. Unstable angina
   C. Cardiac sudden death
   D. Silent ischemia
   E. Postinfarction angina
IV. Extent of coronary atherosclerosis
V. Others
   A. History of hypertension
   B. History of congestive heart failure
   C. Cardiomegaly on chest x-ray
   D. ECG abnormalities
      1. Ventricular arrhythmias
      2. Conduction defects
      3. Abnormal signal averaged ECG
      4. Inducible sustained monomorphic ventricular tachycardia during electrophysiologic testing
   E. Tobacco use
   F. Diabetes mellitus
   G. Age > 70
   H. Female sex
   I. Anterior myocardia

From: Pasternak RC, Braunwald E, Sobel BE. In Braunwald E, et al, editors: *Heart disease: a textbook of cardiovascular medicine*, ed 4. Philadelphia, 1992, W. B. Saunders, p. 1267.

I-18 PSEUDOINFARCTION ECG PATTERNS

  I. Myocardial replacement
     A. Tumor
     B. Abscess
     C. Amyloid disease
     D. Pseudohypertrophic muscular dystrophy
     E. Sarcoid involving the heart
     F. Friedreich's ataxia
     G. Muscular dystrophy
 II. Nonmyocardial replacement
     A. Anatomic factors
        1. Emphysema
        2. Pneumothorax
     B. Inflammatory conditions
        1. Myocarditis
        2. Pericarditis
III. Depolarization abnormalities
     A. IHSS
     B. WPW syndrome
     C. LBBB, LAFB
 IV. Right ventricular hypertrophy
     A. Cor pulmonale
     B. Mitral stenosis
  V. Left ventricular disease
     A. Left ventricular hypertrophy
     B. Congestive cardiomyopathy
     C. Left ventricular aneurysm
 VI. Arrhythmias
     A. Ventricular tachycardia
     B. Electronic pacing of right ventricle
VII. Congestive cardiomyopathy
VIII. Hyperkalemia
 IX. Intracranial hemorrhage
  X. Trauma
 XI. Early repolarization pattern
XII. Hypothermia

IHSS = idiopathic hypertrophic subaortic stenosis
WPW = Wolff-Parkinson-White
LBBB = left bundle branch block
LAFB = left anterior fascicular block

Modified from: Fisch C. In Braunwald E, et al, editors: *Heart disease: a textbook of cardiovascular medicine*, ed 4. Philadelphia, 1992, W. B. Saunders, pp. 116-153.

I-19 CAUSES OF SUDDEN, NONTRAUMATIC DEATH

I. Cardiac
   A. Atherosclerotic coronary artery disease
   B. Stokes-Adams syndrome
   C. Valvular heart disease
      1. Aortic stenosis
      2. Mitral valve prolapse
   D. Myocarditis
   E. Acute pericardial tamponade
   F. Primary myocardial disease
   G. Congestive heart disease
   H. Prolonged Q-T interval syndrome
   I. Drug effects
      1. Hypokalemia
      2. Digitalis
      3. Quinidine and other type I antiarrhythmics
      4. Tricyclic antidepressants
      5. Cocaine
   J. Anomalous conduction pathways
      1. Wolff-Parkinson-White
      2. Lown-Ganong-Levin
   K. Conduction system disease

II. Pulmonary
   A. Cor pulmonale
      1. Acute
      2. Chronic
   B. Status asthmaticus
   C. Asphyxia
      1. Cafe coronary

III. Extracardiac
   A. Dissecting aortic aneurysm
   B. Exsanguinating hemorrhage
   C. Cerebrovascular accident

IV. Miscellaneous
   A. Sudden infant death syndrome
   B. Acute pancreatitis
   C. Unexplained

I-20 RISK FACTORS FOR ANTICOAGULATION

   I. Pre-existing coagulation defect
  II. Ulcerative lesion in the GI tract (peptic ulcer, ulcerative colitis)
 III. Salicylate therapy
 IV. Old age
  V. Poor patient compliance
 VI. Pregnancy
VII. Bacterial endocarditis
VIII. Liver disease
 IX. Advanced retinopathy
  X. Malignant hypertension
 XI. Recent CVA or intracranial process
XII. Unsteady gait

I-21 ETIOLOGIC CLASSIFICATION OF CARDIOMYOPATHIES

I. Primary myocardial involvement
   A. Idiopathic (D,R,H)
   B. Familial (D,H)
   C. Eosinophilic endomyocardial disease (R)
   D. Endomyocardial fibrosis (R)
II. Secondary myocardial involvement
   A. Infective (D)
      1. Viral myocarditis
      2. Bacterial myocarditis
      3. Fungal myocarditis
      4. Protozoal myocarditis
      5. Metazoal myocarditis
   B. Metabolic (D)
   C. Familial storage disease (D,R)
      1. Glycogen storage disease
      2. Mucopolysaccharidoses
   D. Deficiency (D)
      1. Electrolytes
      2. Nutritional
   E. Connective tissue disorders (D)
      1. Systemic lupus erythematosus
      2. Polyarteritis nodosa
      3. Rheumatoid arthritis
      4. Scleroderma
      5. Dermatomyositis
   F. Infiltrations and granulomas (R,D)
      1. Amyloidosis
      2. Sarcoidosis
      3. Malignancy
      4. Hemochromatosis
   G. Neuromuscular (D)
      1. Muscular dystrophy
      2. Myotonic dystrophy
      3. Friedreich's ataxia (H,D)
      4. Refsum's disease
   H. Sensitivity and toxic reactions (D)
      1. Alcohol
      2. Radiation
      3. Drugs (daunorubicin)
   I. Peripartum heart disease (D)
   J. Endocardial fibroelastosis (R)
   K. Obesity (D)

Note: The principal clinical manifestation(s) of each etiologic grouping is denoted by D (dilated), R (restrictive), or H (hypertrophic cardiomyopathy).

I-21 ETIOLOGIC CLASSIFICATION OF CARDIOMYOPATHIES (CONTINUED)

Source: Adapted from the WHO/ISFC task force report on the definition and classification of cardiomyopathies. 1980.

Reference: Braunwald E, Isselbacher KJ, Petersdorf RG, Wilson JD, Martin J, Fauci AS, and Root RK, editors: *Harrison's principles of internal medicine,* ed 12. New York, 1991, McGraw-Hill, p. 976.

I-22 CONGESTIVE HEART FAILURE: PRECIPITATING CAUSES

    I. Pulmonary embolism
    II. Myocardial infarction
    III. Arrhythmias
    IV. Increasingly severe hypertension
    V. Noncompliance with medications
       A. Digitalis
       B. Diuretics
    VI. Excess dietary sodium
    VII. Excess amounts of intravenous fluids
    VIII. Drugs
       A. Propranolol and other beta blockers
       B. Cardiotoxic drugs
          1. Daunorubicin
       C. NSAIDs
       D. Antiarrhythmics (disopyramide)
       E. Corticosteroids
       F. Androgens and estrogens
       G. Tricyclic psychotropic drugs (e.g., nortriptyline)
       H. Cocaine
    IX. Pregnancy
    X. High output states with increased metabolic demands
       A. Fever
       B. Hyperthyroidism
       C. Anemia
       D. AV fistula
       E. Infections
       F. Paget's disease
    XI. Rheumatic and other forms of myocarditis
    XII. Alcohol
    XIII. Infective endocarditis
    XIV. Hypothyroidism
    XV. Renal failure

I-23 REVERSIBLE CAUSES OF CONGESTIVE HEART FAILURE

  I. Anemia
 II. Hyperthyroidism/Hypothyroidism
III. Atrial myxoma
 IV. Arteriovenous fistula
  V. Surgically correctable valvular heart disease
 VI. Surgically correctable congenital heart disease
VII. Cardiac arrhythmias in an otherwise normal heart
VIII. Thiamine deficiency
 IX. Alcohol
  X. Obesity
 XI. Paget's disease

I-24 POTENTIAL LIFE-THREATENING COMPLICATIONS OF ACUTE MYOCARDIAL INFARCTION

  I. Ventricular arrhythmias (ventricular tachycardia, ventricular fibrillation, or asystole)
 II. Extremely rapid atrial arrhythmias in association with extensive myocardial infarction (atrial flutter or atrial fibrillation)
III. Heart block (second- or third-degree)
 IV. Marked bradycardia
  V. Loss of atrial contribution to cardiac contraction (atrioventricular junctional rhythm)
 VI. Infarction $\geq$ 40% of left ventricle
VII. Extensive right ventricular infarction
VIII. Acute and severe mitral regurgitation
 IX. Severe pulmonary edema
  X. Rupture of the heart
 XI. Systemic and/or pulmonary emboli
XII. Cardiogenic shock
XIII. Infarct extension

Modified from: Wyngaarden JB, Smith LH Jr, Bennett JC, editors: *Cecil textbook of medicine*, ed 19. Philadelphia, 1988, W. B. Saunders, p. 336.

I-25 TYPES OF HYPERTENSION

I. Systolic and diastolic hypertension
  A. Primary, essential, or idiopathic
  B. Secondary
    1. Renal
      a. Renal parenchymal disease
        (1) Acute glomerulonephritis
        (2) Chronic nephritis
        (3) Polycystic disease
        (4) Connective tissue diseases
        (5) Diabetic nephropathy
        (6) Hydronephrosis
      b. Renovascular
      c. Renin-producing tumors
      d. Renoprival
      e. Primary sodium retention (Liddle's syndrome, Gordon's syndrome)
    2. Endocrine
      a. Acromegaly
      b. Hypothyroidism
      c. Hypercalcemia
      d. Hyperthyroidism
      e. Adrenal
        (1) Cortical
          (a) Cushing's syndrome
          (b) Primary aldosteronism
          (c) Congenital adrenal hyperplasia
        (2) Medullary: pheochromocytoma
      f. Extra-adrenal chromaffin tumors
      g. Carcinoid
      h. Exogenous hormones
        (1) Estrogen
        (2) Glucocorticoid
        (3) Mineralocorticoids: licorice, carbenexolone
        (4) Sympathomimetics
        (5) Tyramine-containing foods and MAO inhibitors
    3. Coarctation of the aorta
    4. Pregnancy-induced hypertension
    5. Neurological disorders
      a. Increased intracranial pressure
        (1) Brain tumor
        (2) Encephalitis
        (3) Respiratory acidosis: lung or CNS disease
      b. Quadriplegia
      c. Acute porphyria
      d. Familial dysautonomia (Riley-Day)

I-25 TYPES OF HYPERTENSION (CONTINUED)

   e. Lead poisoning
   f. Guillain-Barré syndrome
  6. Acute stress, including surgery
   a. Psychogenic hyperventilation
   b. Hypoglycemia
   c. Burns
   d. Pancreatitis
   e. Alcohol withdrawal
   f. Sickle cell crisis
   g. Postresuscitation
   h. Postoperative
  7. Increased intravascular volume
  8. Drugs and other substances
 II. Systolic hypertension
  A. Increased cardiac output
   1. Aortic valvular regurgitation
   2. AV fistula, patent ductus
   3. Thyrotoxicosis
   4. Paget's disease of bone
   5. Beriberi
   6. Hyperkinetic circulation
  B. Rigidity of aorta

Modified from: Kaplan NM. In Braunwald E, et al, editors: *Heart disease, a textbook of cardiovascular medicine,* ed 4. Philadelphia, 1992, W. B. Saunders, p. 820.

I-26 FACTORS INDICATING AN ADVERSE PROGNOSIS IN HYPERTENSION

  I. Black race
  II. Youth
  III. Male
  IV. Persistent diastolic pressure > 115 mm Hg
  V. Smoking
  VI. Diabetes mellitus
  VII. Hypercholesterolemia
 VIII. Obesity
  IX. Evidence of end organ damage
  A. Cardiac
   1. Cardiac enlargement
   2. ECG changes of ischemic or left ventricular strain
   3. Myocardial infarction
   4. Congestive heart failure
  B. Eyes
   1. Retinal exudates and hemorrhages
   2. Papilledema

I-26 FACTORS INDICATING AN ADVERSE PROGNOSIS IN HYPERTENSION (CONTINUED)

  C. Renal: impaired renal function
  D. Nervous system: cerebrovascular accident
 X. High-renin hypertension

Modified from: Williams GH, et al: In Braunwald E, Isselbacher KJ, Petersdorf RG, Wilson JD, Martin J, Fauci AS, Root RK, editors: *Harrison's principles of internal medicine*, ed 12. New York, 1991, McGraw-Hill, p. 1004.

I-27 ETIOLOGY OF SYNCOPE, WEAKNESS, AND FAINTNESS

  I. Circulatory (deficient quantity of blood to the brain)
    A. Inadequate vasoconstrictor mechanisms
      1. Vasovagal (vasodepression)
      2. Postural hypotension
      3. Primary autonomic insufficiency
      4. Sympathectomy (pharmacologic due to antihypertensive medications such as Aldomet and hydralazine, or surgical)
      5. Diseases of central and peripheral nervous systems, including autonomic nerves
      6. Carotid sinus syncope (see also "Bradyarrhythmias," below)
      7. Hyperbradykininemia
    B. Hypovolemia
      1. Blood loss — gastrointestinal hemorrhage
      2. Addison's disease
    C. Mechanical reduction of venous return
      1. Valsalva maneuver
      2. Cough (posttussive)
      3. Micturition
      4. Atrial myxoma, ball valve thrombus
    D. Reduced cardiac output
      1. Obstruction to left ventricular outflow: Aortic stenosis, hypertrophic subaortic stenosis
      2. Obstruction to pulmonary flow: Pulmonic stenosis, primary pulmonary hypertension, pulmonary embolism
      3. Myocardial: Massive myocardial infarction with pump failure
      4. Pericardial: Cardiac tamponade
    E. Arrhythmias
      1. Bradyarrhythmias
        a. Atrioventricular (AV) block (2nd and 3rd degree), with Stokes-Adams attacks

I-27 ETIOLOGY OF SYNCOPE, WEAKNESS, AND FAINTNESS (CONTINUED)

 b. Ventricular asystole
 c. Sinus bradycardia, sinoatrial block, sinus arrest
 d. Carotid sinus syncope (see also inadequate vasoconstrictor mechanisms, above)
 e. Glossopharyngeal neuralgia (and other painful states)
 2. Tachyarrhythmias
 a. Episodic ventricular tachycardia with or without associated bradyarrhythmias
 b. Supraventricular tachycardia without AV block
II. Other causes of weakness and episodic disturbances of consciousness
 A. Altered state of blood to the brain
 1. Hypoxia
 2. Anemia
 3. Diminished carbon dioxide due to hyperventilation (faintness common, syncope seldom occurs)
 4. Hypoglycemia (episodic weakness common, faintness occasional, syncope rare)
 B. Cerebral
 1. Cerebrovascular disturbances (TIA's, etc.)
 a. Extracranial vascular insufficiency (vertebral-basilar, carotid)
 b. Diffuse spasm of cerebral arterioles (hypertensive encephalopathy)
 2. Emotional disturbances, anxiety attacks, and hysterical seizures

Modified from: Ruskin J, Martin J. In Braunwald E, Isselbacher KJ, Petersdorf RG, Wilson JD, Martin J, Fauci AS, Root RK, editors: *Harrison's principles of internal medicine*, ed 12. New York, 1991, McGraw-Hill, p. 134.

I-28 CLASSIFICATION OF PERICARDITIS

I. Clinical classification
  A. Acute pericarditis (< 6 weeks)
     1. Fibrinous
     2. Effusive (or bloody)
  B. Subacute pericarditis (6 weeks to 6 months)
     1. Constrictive
     2. Effusive-constrictive
  C. Chronic pericarditis (> 6 months)
     1. Constrictive
     2. Effusive
     3. Adhesive (nonconstrictive)
II. Etiologic classification
  A. Infectious pericarditis
     1. Viral
     2. Pyogenic
     3. Tuberculous
     4. Mycotic
     5. Other infections (syphilitic, parasitic)
  B. Noninfectious pericarditis
     1. Acute myocardial infarction
     2. Uremia
     3. Neoplasia
        a. Primary tumors (benign or malignant)
        b. Tumors metastatic to pericardium
     4. Myxedema
     5. Cholesterol
     6. Chylopericardium
     7. Trauma
        a. Penetrating chest wall
        b. Nonpenetrating
     8. Aortic aneurysm (with leakage into pericardial sac)
     9. Postirradiation
    10. Associated with atrial septal defect
    11. Associated with severe chronic anemia
    12. Infectious mononucleosis
    13. Familial Mediterranean fever
    14. Familial pericarditis
        a. Mulibrey nanism*
    15. Sarcoidosis
    16. Acute idiopathic
  C. Pericarditis presumably related to hypersensitivity of autoimmunity
     1. Rheumatic fever
     2. Collagen vascular disease
        a. Systemic lupus erythematosus

I-28 CLASSIFICATION OF PERICARDITIS (CONTINUED)

            b. Rheumatoid arthritis
            c. Scleroderma
        3. Drug-induced
            a. Procainamide
            b. Hydralazine
            c. Other
        4. Postcardiac injury
            a. Postmyocardial infarction (Dressler's syndrome)
            b. Postpericardiotomy

*An autosomal recessive syndrome, characterized by growth failure, muscle hypotonia, hepatomegaly, ocular changes, enlarged cerebral ventricles, mental retardation, and chronic constrictive pericarditis.

Source: Braunwald E. In Braunwald E, Isselbacher KJ, Petersdorf RG, Wilson JD, Martin J, Fauci AS, Root RK, editors: *Harrison's principles of internal medicine*, ed 12. New York, 1991, McGraw-Hill, p. 981.

I-29 ETIOLOGY OF CHRONIC CONSTRICTIVE PERICARDITIS

   I. Unknown
  II. Following idiopathic pericarditis
 III. Specific infection
       A. Bacterial
       B. Tuberculosis (50% to 65% of treated pericarditis)
       C. Fungal disease (rare): histoplasmosis, coccidioidomycosis
       D. Viral disease, esp. Coxsackie B_3
       E. Parasitic disease: amebiasis, echinococcosis
  IV. Connective tissue disease: rheumatoid arthritis, lupus erythematosus
   V. Neoplastic disease
       A. Primary mesothelioma
       B. Secondary lymphoma, bronchogenic carcinoma, breast
  VI. Trauma
       A. Blunt or penetrating
       B. Surgical (rare)
 VII. Radiation therapy
VIII. Uremic
  IX. Hereditary (mulibrey nanism — Finland)

I-30 CLINICAL FEATURES OF CONSTRICTIVE PERICARDITIS (137 CASES)*

I. Symptoms
  A. Effort dyspnea — 89.8%
  B. Chest pain — 24%†
  C. RUQ or epigastric pain — 10.9%
  D. Effort syncope — 4 cases
  E. Orthopnea, paroxysmal nocturnal dyspnea — 3 cases
II. Physical findings
  A. Atrial fibrillation — 27%
  B. Cervical veins engorged. Venous pressure 15-44 cm H_2O
  C. Liver enlarged — 134 cases
  D. Ascites — 77.4%
  E. Peripheral edema — 61%
  F. Pleural effusion — 47%
  G. Paradoxical pulse — 29%
  H. Early diastolic heart sound — 20 cases

*Reference: Wychulis, et al. *J Thorac Cardiovasc Surg* 62:608, 1971
†Most studies do not report so high a prevalence of chest pain. Hirschmann. *Am Heart J* 96:111, 1978.

I-31 ETIOLOGY OF PERICARDIAL EFFUSION

I. Serous
   A. Congestive heart failure
   B. Hypoalbuminemia
   C. Irradiation
   D. Viral pericarditis
   E. Tuberculous pericarditis
   F. Bacterial pericarditis
   G. Dressler's syndrome
   H. Chemotherapeutic agents
   I. Myxedema
II. Blood (hematocrit > 10%)
   A. Iatrogenic
      1. Cardiac operation
      2. Cardiac catheterization
      3. Trauma (penetrating and nonpenetrating)
      4. Anticoagulant agents
      5. Chemotherapeutic agents
   B. Neoplasm
   C. Trauma
   D. Acute myocardial infarction
   E. Cardiac rupture
   F. Rupture of ascending aorta or major pulmonary artery
   G. Coagulopathy
   H. Uremia
III. Lymph or chyle
   A. Neoplasm
   B. Iatrogenic
      1. Cardiothoracic surgery
   C. Congenital
   D. Idiopathic ("primary chylopericardium")
   E. Nonneoplastic obstruction of thoracic duct

Modified from: Shabetai R. In Wyngaarden JB, Smith LH Jr, Bennett JC editors: *Cecil textbook of medicine*, ed 19. Philadelphia, 1988, W. B. Saunders, p. 343.

I-32 COMMON ETIOLOGIES OF CARDIAC TAMPONADE

Disorder	1980 %	1988 %
Malignant disease	32	58
Idiopathic pericarditis	14	14
Uremia	9	14
Acute cardiac infarction (receiving heparin)	9	
Diagnostic procedures with cardiac perforation	7.5	
Bacterial	7.5	5
Tuberculosis	5	1
Radiation	4	
Myxedema	4	
Dissecting aortic aneurysm	4	
Postpericardiotomy syndrome	2	
Systemic lupus erythematosus	2	2
Cardiomyopathy (receiving anticoagulants)	2	6

Modified from: Lorell BH. In Braunwald E, et al, editors: *Heart disease, a textbook of cardiovascular medicine*, ed 4. Philadelphia, 1992, W. B. Saunders, p. 1476

I-33 PREDISPOSING FACTORS TO CHRONIC PULMONARY HYPERTENSION AND COR PULMONALE

I. Hypoxic vasoconstriction
   A. Chronic bronchitis and emphysema, cystic fibrosis
   B. Chronic hypoventilation
      1. Obesity
      2. Sleep apnea
      3. Neuromuscular disease
      4. Chest wall dysfunction
      5. Primary or idiopathic alveolar hypoventilation ("Ondine's curse")
   C. High-altitude dwelling and chronic mountain sickness

II. Occlusion of the pulmonary vascular bed
   A. Pulmonary thromboembolism, parasitic ova, tumor emboli
   B. Primary pulmonary hypertension
   C. Pulmonary venocclusive disease
   D. Fibrosing mediastinitis, mediastinal tumor
   E. Pulmonary angiitis from systemic disease
      1. Collagen vascular diseases
      2. Drug-induced lung disease
      3. Necrotizing and granulomatous arteritis

III Parenchymal disease with loss of vascular surface area
   A. Bullous emphysema, α_1-antiproteinase deficiency
   B. Diffuse bronchiectasis, cystic fibrosis
   C. Diffuse interstitial disease
      1. Pneumoconioses
      2. Sarcoid, idiopathic pulmonary fibrosis, histiocytosis X
      3. Tuberculosis, chronic fungal infection
      4. ARDS
      5. Collagen vascular disease (immune lung disease)
      6. Hypersensitivity pneumonitis

IV. Cardiac disease
   A. Acquired disorders of the left side of the heart causing pulmonary venous hypertension
      1. Left ventricular failure
      2. Mitral valve disease
      3. Left atrial myxoma
      4. Decrease in left ventricular compliance
   B. Congenital heart disease
      1. Pretricuspid
      2. Posttricuspid

Modified from: Hurst JW. In Hurst JW, Rackley CE, Sonnenblick EH, Wenger NK, editors: *The heart,* ed 7. New York, 1990, McGraw-Hill, p. 1220.

I-34 PULMONARY VALVULAR INSUFFICIENCY

I. Congenital
   A. With tetralogy of Fallot
   B. With Eisenmenger's syndrome
   C. With Marfan's syndrome
   D. Isolated
   E. With patent ductus arteriosus
   F. With idiopathic dilation of the pulmonary artery
II. Acquired as a result of other congenital heart disease.
   A. Following operation on the stenotic pulmonary valve
   B. With pulmonary hypertension related to patent ductus arteriosus, atrial septal defect, or ventricular septal defect
III. As a result of acquired heart disease
   A. With idiopathic or thromboembolic pulmonary hypertension
   B. With mitral stenosis
   C. With bacterial endocarditis
   D. With rheumatic fever
   E. With syphilis
   F. With carcinoid syndrome
   G. With aneurysm of the pulmonary artery (often syphilitic)
   H. With pulmonary hypertension and chronic lung disease

I-35 FACTORS PREDISPOSING TO THROMBOEMBOLISM

I. Heart disease, especially
   A. Myocardial infarction
   B. Atrial fibrillation
   C. Cardiomyopathy
   D. Congestive heart failure
II. Postoperative state, especially operations on abdomen or pelvis, splenectomy, and orthopedic procedures on lower extremities
III. Pregnancy and parturition
IV. Neoplastic disease
V. Polycythemia
VI. Prolonged immobilization
VII. Hemorrhage
VIII. Fractures, especially of the hip
IX. Obesity
X. Varicose veins
XI. Prior history of thromboembolic disease
XII. Certain drugs: oral contraceptives, estrogens
XIII. Following cerebrovascular accidents
XIV. Abnormal blood flow
XV. Myeloproliferative disorders with thrombocytosis
XVI. Antithrombin III deficiency
XVII. Protein C deficiency, protein S deficiency
XVIII. Abnormal fibrinolysis

I-36 DIGITALIS INTOXICATION

I. Patients with increased risk of digitalis intoxication
   A. Renal insufficiency or failure
   B. Malabsorption
   C. Elderly patients
   D. Obese patients
   E. Electrolyte imbalance (decreased K^+, increased Ca^{2+}, decreased Mg^{2+})
   F. Liver disease (digitoxin only)
   G. Thyroid disease (hypothyroidism)
   H. Pulmonary disease
   I. Drugs (quinidine, verapamil, diltiazem, amiodarone, and procainamide)

II. *Diagnosis of digitalis intoxication
   A. Symptoms: diarrhea, anorexia, nausea, emesis, visual disturbances
   B. Arrhythmias
   C. Digitalis dose excessive for body weight
      1. Usual maintenance dose of digoxin is 3 μg/kg
   D. Digitalis dose excessive in the presence of impaired renal function
   E. Increased serum digitalis glycoside levels
   F. Improvement in items A, B, and E after discontinuation of and/or readjustment in glycoside dosage

*These findings are not always present

I-37 ASSESSMENT OF CARDIOVASCULAR RISK IN PATIENTS BEING CONSIDERED FOR SURGERY

Risk factor present	Points
I. History	
A. Age > 70	5
B. Myocardial infarction previous 6 mo.	10
II. Physical examination	
A. Aortic stenosis	3
B. Signs of congestive heart failure, S_3 gallop, jugular venous distention	11
III. Cardiac rhythm	
A. Premature ventricular contractions	7
B. Rhythm other than normal sinus	7
IV. Miscellaneous	
A. Emergent procedure	4
B. Intrathoracic/intra-abdominal procedure	3
C. ↑BUN, ↓ serum K^+, ↓ arterial pO_2	3
Total possible points	53

V. Assessment of Risk

0	-	5 points	Minimal	(Grade I)
6	-	12 points	Minimal—Moderate	(Grade II)
13	-	25 points	Moderate to Severe	(Grade III)
	>	26 points	Prohibitive	(Grade IV)

Reference: Goldman L. *New Engl J Med* 297:845, 1977

I-38 CLASSIFICATION OF ANTIARRHYTHMIC DRUGS ACCORDING TO THEIR MECHANISM OF ACTION

Class	Action	Drugs
I.	Fast sodium channel blockade	
	A. Reduce V_{max}, prolong action potential duration	Quinidine, procainamide, disopyramide
	B. Do not change V_{max}, shorten action potential duration	Tocainide, mexiletine, phenytoin, lidocaine, probably moricizine
	C. Reduce V_{max}, primarily slow conduction: can prolong refractoriness	Flecainide, encainide, propafenone
II.	Beta-adrenergic blockade	Esmolol, propranolol, timolol, metoprolol, sotalol, others
III.	Block potassium channels, prolong repolarization	Sotalol, amiodarone, bretylium, N-acetyl-procainamide
IV.	Calcium channel blockade	Verapamil, diltiazem, nifedpine, others

Adapted from: Zipes DP. In Braunwald E, et al, editors: *Heart disease, a textbook of cardiovascular medicine*, ed 4. Philadelphia, 1992, W. B. Saunders, p. 628.

I-39 DEFINITE INDICATIONS FOR IMPLANTED PACEMAKER

I. Complete heart block, permanent or intermittent, with any one of the following complications:
   A. Symptomatic bradycardia
   B. Congestive heart failure
   C. Conditions that require treatment with drugs that suppress ventricular escape rhythms
   D. Asystole $\geq$ 3 seconds or ventricular rate < 40 per minute.
   E. Mental confusion that clears with pacing

II. Patients with complete heart block or advanced second-degree AV block that persists after myocardial infarction

III. Chronic bi- or trifascicular block with intermittent complete heart block or type II second-degree AV block associated with symptomatic bradycardia.

IV. Sinus node dysfunction with documented symptomatic bradycardia

V. Hypersensitive carotid sinus syndrome with recurrent syncope and asystole > 3 seconds provoked by minimal carotid sinus pressure

VI. Symptomatic supraventricular tachycardia that does not respond to medical treatment.

Reference: Barold SS, Zipes DP. In Braunwald E, et al, editors: *Heart disease, a textbook of cardiovascular medicine,* ed 4. Philadelphia, 1992, W. B. Saunders, p. 728.

I-40 INDICATIONS FOR CLINICAL ELECTROPHYSIOLOGICAL STUDIES — ENDOCARDIAL ELECTRICAL STIMULATION

I. To evaluate mechanism, site, and extent of arrhythmia and/or conduction defect.
   A. Sick sinus syndrome
   B. Pre-excitation syndrome
   C. Supraventricular tachycardia
   D. Distinguish between supraventricular arrhythmias with aberration and ventricular arrhythmia
   E. Type I AV block with bundle branch block
   F. Type II AV block with normal QRS
   G. Bifascicular block occurring in acute myocardial infarction

II. To search for a cause for syncope
   A. Evaluate sinus node function
   B. Evaluate AV node function
   C. Evaluate function of His-Purkinje system
   D. Evaluate functional characteristics of anomalous AV connections
   E. Provoke arrhythmias
      1. Supraventricular tachycardia
      2. Atrial flutter or fibrillation
      3. Ventricular tachycardia

III. To evaluate therapy
   A. Drug therapy
      1. Prevent inducible arrhythmias
      2. Measure conduction and refractoriness in anomalous AV connections
      3. Evaluate adverse effects
         a. Sinus node function
         b. AV node function
         c. His-Purkinje system
         d. Effect on device function
   B. Surgical therapy
      1. Preoperative endocardial catheter mapping
         a. Location of anomalous AV connections
         b. Location of VT circuit
         c. Need for concomitant pacemaker implantation
      2. Postoperative evaluation
         a. Presence of anomalous AV connections
         b. Arrhythmia inducible
   C. AICD therapy
      1. Preoperative evaluation

I-40 INDICATIONS FOR CLINICAL ELECTROPHYSIOLOGICAL STUDIES — ENDOCARDIAL ELECTRICAL STIMULATION (CONTINUED)

        a. Determine that VT or VF is inducible
        b. Determine that VT or VF is drug resistant
        c. Determine need for concomitant pacemaker implantation

2. Intraoperative evaluation
    a. Determine equality of right or left ventricular sensing electrograms
    b. Determine quality of patch electrograms for the probability density function.
    c. Determine defibrillation thresholds
    d. Induce clinical arrhythmia to test sensing and termination of ventricular arrhythmias by the AICD

3. Postoperative evaluation
    a. Induce VT or VF to test the performance of the AICD
    b. Acquaint the patient with the symptoms during AICD discharge

  D. Pacemaker therapy
    1. Evaluate condition for suitability for pacemaker therapy
      a. Supraventricular tachycardia-reciprocation in the AV node
      b. Supraventricular tachycardia-reciprocation in anomalous AV connections
    2. Determine the information needed to select pacemaker type and parameters

IV. To apply ablation therapy
  A. Posterior septal anomalous AV connections
  B. AV node
  C. Ventricular tachycardia

AICD = automatic implantable cardioverter defibrillator; VT = ventricular tachycardia; VF = ventricular fibrillation.

Reference: Bigger JT. In Wyngaarden JB, Smith LH Jr, Bennett JC editors: *Cecil textbook of medicine*, ed 19. Philadelphia, 1988, W. B. Saunders, p. 234.

I-41 NBG PACEMAKER CODE (1987)

Code Positions*

I† Chamber paced	II† Chamber sensed	III Response to sensing	IV Programmable functions; rate modulation	V Antitachyarrhythmia functions
V—ventricle	V—ventricle	T—triggers pacing	P—programmable rate and/or output	P—antitachy-arrhythmia
A—atrium	A—atrium	I—inhibits pacing	M—multiprogramma-bility of rate, output, sensitivity, etc.	S—shock
D—double	D—double	D—triggers and inhibits pacing	C—communicating functions (telemetry)	D—dual (P + S)
O—none	O—none	O—none	R—rare modulation	O—none
			O—none	

C
O
D
E

L
E
T
T
E
R
S

*Positions I-III are used exclusively for antibradyarrhythmia pacing.
†Manufacturers often use "S" for single-chamber (A or V).

Reference: Mond, SJ. In Hurst JW, Rackley CE, Sonnenblick EH, Wenger NK, editors: *The heart*, ed 7. New York, 1990, McGraw-Hill, p. 570.

I-42 CAUSES OF SHOCK AND INITIATING MECHANISMS

I. Hypovolemic shock
  A. Hemorrhagic (e.g., trauma, gastrointestinal hemorrhage)
  B. Hypovolemic, nonhemorrhagic
    1. External fluid loss (e.g., vomiting, diarrhea, polyuria, burns)
    2. Internal extravascular sequestration (e.g., peritonitis, pancreatitis)

II. Cardiogenic shock
  A. Acute myocardial infarction
    1. Loss of critical muscle mass (e.g., large anterior wall infarction)
    2. Acute mechanical lesion (e.g., ventricular septal rupture, mitral insufficiency)
    3. Acute right ventricular infarction
    4. Left ventricular free wall rupture
    5. Left ventricular aneurysm
  B. Valvular heart disease
    1. Critical valvular stenosis (e.g., aortic or mitral stenosis)
    2. Severe valvular insufficiency (e.g., acute aortic or mitral insufficiency)
  C. Nonvalvular obstructive cardiac lesions
    1. Atrial myxoma or ball-valve thrombus
    2. Cardiac tamponade
    3. Restrictive cardiomyopathy (e.g., amyloid)
    4. Constrictive pericardial disorder
  D. Nonischemic myopathic processes
    1. Fulminant myocarditis
    2. Physiologic depressants (e.g., acidosis, hypoxia)
    3. Pharmacologic depressants (e.g., calcium channel blockers)
    4. Pathophysiologic depressants (e.g., myocardial depressant factor)
  E. Dysrhythmias
    1. Severe bradyarrhythmias (e.g., high-degree AV block)
    2. Tachyarrhythmias
      a. Ventricular (e.g., ventricular tachycardia)
      b. Supraventricular (e.g., atrial fibrillation or flutter with rapid ventricular response)

III. Vascular obstructive shock
  A. Massive pulmonary embolism
  B. Tension pneumothorax
  C. Excessive positive-pressure ventilation
  D. Aortic dissection

I-42 CAUSES OF SHOCK AND INITIATING MECHANISMS (CONTINUED)

IV. Distributive shock and miscellaneous
   A. Sepsis
   B. Anaphylaxis
   C. Massive tissue injury (e.g., crush)
   D. Prolonged ischemia/hypoxia
   E. Neurogenic shock
   F. Endocrine disorders
      1. Addisonian crisis
      2. Profound hypothyroidism
   G. Drug or toxin induced

Reference: Ferguson DW. In Wyngaarden JB, Smith LH Jr, Bennett JC editors: *Cecil textbook of medicine*, ed 19. Philadelphia, 1988, W. B. Saunders, p. 216.

I-43 CONTRAINDICATIONS TO THROMBOLYTIC THERAPY

I. Absolute contraindications
   A. Active internal bleeding
   B. Suspected aortic dissection
   C. Prolonged (>10 min) or traumatic cardiopulmonary resuscitation
   D. Recent head trauma or known intracranial neoplasm
   E. Diabetic hemorrhagic retinopathy or other hemorrhagic ophthalmic condition
   F. Known or suspected pregnancy
   G. Previous allergic reaction to a thrombolytic agent
   H. Recorded blood pressure higher than 200/120 mm Hg
   I. History of hemorrhagic cerebrovascular accident
   J. Trauma or surgery in past 2 weeks that could be source of rebleeding

II. Relative contraindications or other considerations*
   A. History of chronic, severe hypertension with or without drug therapy
   B. Active peptic ulcer
   C. History of cerebrovascular event or spinal surgery
   D. Known bleeding diathesis (severe thrombocytopenia, coagulopathies) or current use of anticoagulants
   E. Predisposition to bleeding due to polycystic kidney, gastrointestinal arteriovenous malformation, vascular tumors, or severe liver disease
   F. Use of streptokinase (Kabikinase, Streptase) or APSAC (anistreplase [Eminase]), or streptococcal infection within past 6 to 9 mo
   G. Old coronary artery bypass graft to infarct-related artery
   H. Neoplastic disease
   I. Any condition likely to affect 1-year survival
   J. ST-segment elevation with ongoing ischemic chest pain for more than 6 hr
   K. Clinical evidence of reinfarction days after administration of thrombolytic therapy
   L. Unstable angina.

*Therapy should be considered on a case-by-case analysis of risk versus benefit.

Modified from: Selig MD. *Postgraduate Med* 92(1):211, 1992.

I-44 BACTERIAL ENDOCARDITIS PROPHYLAXIS

I. Cardiac conditions
   A. Endocarditis prophylaxis recommended
      1. Prosthetic cardiac valves, including bioprosthetic and homograft valves
      2. Previous bacterial endocarditis, even in the absence of heart disease
      3. Most congenital cardiac malformations
      4. Rheumatic and other acquired valvular dysfunction, even after valvular surgery
      5. Hypertrophic cardiomyopathy
      6. Mitral valve prolapse with valvular regurgitation
   B. Endocarditis prophylaxis not recommended
      1. Isolated secundum atrial septal defect
      2. Surgical repair without residua beyond 6 mo of secundum atrial septal defect, ventricular septal defect, or patent ductus arteriosus
      3. Previous coronary artery bypass graft surgery
      4. Mitral valve prolapse without valvular regurgitation†
      5. Physiologic, functional, or innocent heart murmurs
      6. Previous Kawasaki disease without valvular dysfunction
      7. Previous rheumatic fever without valvular dysfunction
      8. Cardiac pacemakers and implanted defibrillators
II. Dental or surgical procedures
   A. Endocarditis prophylaxis recommended
      1. Dental procedures known to induce gingival or mucosal bleeding, including professional cleaning
      2. Tonsillectomy and/or adenoidectomy
      3. Surgical operations that involve intestinal or respiratory mucosa
      4. Bronchoscopy with a rigid bronchoscope
      5. Sclerotherapy for esophageal varices
      6. Esophageal dilatation
      7. Gallbladder surgery
      8. Cystoscopy
      9. Urethral dilatation
      10. Urethral catheterization if urinary tract infection is present‡
      11. Urinary tract surgery if urinary tract infection is present‡
      12. Prostatic surgery
      13. Incision and drainage of infected tissue‡
      14. Vaginal hysterectomy
      15. Vaginal delivery in the presence of infection‡

I-44   BACTERIAL ENDOCARDITIS PROPHYLAXIS (CONTINUED)

B. Endocarditis prophylaxis not recommended§
   1. Dental procedures not likely to induce gingival bleeding, such as simple adjustment of orthodontic appliances or fillings above the gum line
   2. Injection of local intraoral anesthetic (except intraligamentary injections)
   3. Shedding of primary teeth
   4. Tympanostomy tube insertion
   5. Endotracheal intubation
   6. Bronchoscopy with a flexible bronchoscope, with or without biopsy
   7. Cardiac catheterization
   8. Endoscopy with or without gastrointestinal biopsy
   9. Cesarean section
   10. In the absence of infection for urethral catheterization, dilatation and curettage, uncomplicated vaginal delivery, therapeutic abortion, sterilization procedures, or insertion or removal of intrauterine devices

*This table lists selected conditions but is not meant to be all-inclusive
†Individuals who have a mitral valve prolapse associated with thickening and/or redundancy of the valve leaflets may be at increased risk for bacterial endocarditis, particularly men who are 45 years of age or older.
‡In addition to prophylactic regimen for genitourinary procedures, antibiotic therapy should be directed against the most likely bacterial pathogen.
§In patients who have prosthetic heart valves, a previous history of endocarditis, or surgically constructed systemic-pulmonary shunts or conduits, physicians may choose to administer prophylactic antibiotics even for low-risk procedures that involve the lower respiratory, genitourinary, or gastrointestinal tracts.

Reference: Dajani A.S., et al. JAMA 264(22):2919-22, 1990.

CHAPTER II
ENDOCRINOLOGY—
METABOLISM

II-1 DISORDERS ASSOCIATED WITH HYPOPITUITARISM

I. Primary
  A. Ischemic necrosis of the pituitary
    1. Postpartum (Sheehan's syndrome)
    2. Diabetes mellitus
    3. Other systemic diseases (temporal arteritis, sickle-cell disease and trait, arteriosclerosis, eclampsia)
  B. Pituitary tumors
    1. Primary intrasellar (chromophobe adenoma, craniopharyngioma)
    2. Parasellar (meningioma, optic nerve glioma)
  C. Aneurysm of intracranial internal carotid artery
  D. Pituitary apoplexy (almost always related to a primary pituitary tumor)
  E. Cavernous sinus thrombosis
  F. Infectious disease (tuberculosis, syphilis, malaria, meningitis, fungal disease)
  G. Infiltrative disease (hemochromatosis)
  H. Immunologic (granulomatous or lymphocytic hypophysitis)
  I. Iatrogenic
    1. Irradiation to nasopharynx
    2. Irradiation to sella
    3. Surgical destruction
  J. Primary empty sella syndrome
  K. Metabolic disorders (chronic renal failure)
  L. Idiopathic (frequently monohormonal and occasionally familial)
II. Secondary
  A. Destruction of pituitary stalk
    1. Trauma
    2. Compression by tumor or aneurysm
    3. Iatrogenic (surgical)
  B. Hypothalamic or other central nervous system disease
    1. Inflammatory (sarcoid or other granulomatous disease)
    2. Infiltrative (lipid storage diseases)
    3. Trauma
    4. Toxic (vincristine)
    5. Hormone-induced (glucocorticoids, gonadal steroids)
    6. Tumors (primary, metastatic, lymphomas, leukemia)
    7. Idiopathic (frequently congenital or familial, often restricted to one or two hormones, and may be reversible)
    8. Nutritional (starvation, obesity)
    9. Anorexia nervosa
    10. Psychosocial dwarfism

II-1 DISORDERS ASSOCIATED WITH HYPOPITUITARISM (CONTINUED)

Adapted from: Frohman, L.A.: In *Endocrinology and Metabolism*, Felig P, Baxter JD, Broadus AE and Frohman, L.A. (eds.), ed 2. New York, 1987, McGraw-Hill, p. 274.

II-2 DIFFERENTIAL DIAGNOSIS OF HYPERPROLACTINEMIA

  I. Prolactin-secreting pituitary tumor
 II. Pharmacologic agents
    A. Monoamine synthesis inhibitors (alpha-methyldopa)
    B. Monoamine depletors (reserpine)
    C. Dopamine receptor antagonists (phenothiazines, butyrophenones, thioxanthenes)
    D. Monoamine uptake inhibitors (tricyclic antidepressants)
    E. Estrogens (oral contraceptives)
    F. Narcotics (morphine, heroin)
III. Central nervous system disorders
    A. Inflammatory/infiltrative (sarcoidosis, histiocytosis)
    B. Traumatic (stalk section)
    C. Neoplastic (hypothalamic or parasellar tumors)
 IV. Other
    A. Hypothyroidism
    B. Renal failure
    C. Cirrhosis
    D. Autoimmune or granulomatous hypophysitis
    E. Chest wall diseases
    F. Spinal cord lesions
    G. Empty sella
  V. "Idiopathic hyperprolactinemia"

Adapted from: Frohman LA. In Felig P, Baxter JD, Broadus AE, Frohman LA, editors: *Endocrinology and metabolism*, ed 2. New York, 1987, McGraw-Hill, p. 309.

II-3   CLINICAL FEATURES OF ACROMEGALY

Clinical features	Diagnosis
I. Enlargement of hands, feet, nose, jaw	I. Inappropriately ↑ plasma growth hormone
II. Soft tissue overgrowth	II. Failure of IV glucose to suppress plasma growth hormone
III. Weight gain	
IV. Amenorrhea	III. Abnormal growth hormone response to thyrotropin releasing hormone
V. Decreased libido	
VI. Arthritis	
VII. Hypertrichosis	IV. Hyperglycemia and glucosuria
VIII. Hypertension	
IX. Glucose intolerance	V. ↑ sella turcica (90%)
X. Cardiac arrhythmias	VI. Abnormal CT scan
XI. Visual field defects	
XII. Paresthesias/peripheral neuropathy	
XIII. Carpal tunnel syndrome	

II-4   FEATURES COMMONLY ASSOCIATED WITH THE PRIMARY EMPTY SELLA SYNDROME

	Frequency, %
Females	83.7
Obesity	78.4
Systemic hypertension	30.5
Benign intracranial hypertension (pseudotumor cerebri)	10.5
CSF rhinorrhea	9.7

Reference: Jordan, et al.: The primary empty sella syndrome. *Am J Med* 62:569, 1977.

II-5 PHYSIOLOGICAL CLASSIFICATION OF GALACTORRHEA

I. Failure of normal hypothalamic inhibition of prolactin release
   A. Pituitary stalk section
   B. Drugs (phenothiazines, butyrophenones, methyldopa, tricyclic antidepressants, opiates, reserpine, verapamil)
   C. Central nervous system disease
II. Enhanced prolactin-releasing factor
   A. Hypothyroidism
   B. Sucking reflex and breast trauma
III. Autonomous prolactin release
   A. Pituitary tumors
      1. Prolactin-secreting tumors (Forbes-Albright syndrome)
      2. Mixed growth hormone and prolactin-secreting tumors
      3. Chromophobe adenoma
   B. Ectopic production of human placental lactogen and/or prolactin
      1. Hydatidiform moles and choriocarcinomas
      2. Others (bronchogenic carcinoma and hypernephroma)
IV. Idiopathic (with or without amenorrhea)

Modified from: Wilson JD. In Braunwald E, Isselbacher KJ, Petersdorf RG, Wilson JD, Martin J, Fauci AS, Root RK, editors: *Harrison's principles of internal medicine*, ed 12. New York, 1991, McGraw-Hill, p. 1796.

II-6 DIFFERENTIAL DIAGNOSIS OF THE SYNDROME OF INAPPROPRIATE ANTIDIURESIS (SIADH)

I. Tumors
   A. Bronchogenic carcinoma
   B. Carcinoma of the duodenum
   C. Carcinoma of pancreas
   D. Thymoma
   E. Carcinoma of ureter
   F. Lymphoma
   G. Ewing's sarcoma
   H. Carcinoma of the prostate
   I. Mesothelioma
   J. Carcinoma of the bladder
II. Nonneoplastic diseases
   A. Trauma
   B. Pulmonary disease
      1. Pneumonia, bacterial or viral
      2. Cavitation (aspergillosis)
      3. Tuberculosis
      4. Positive-pressure breathing

II-6 DIFFERENTIAL DIAGNOSIS OF THE SYNDROME OF INAPPROPRIATE ANTIDIURESIS (SIADH) (CONTINUED)

      5. Lung abscess
      6. Asthma
      7. Pneumothorax
      8. Cystic fibrosis

  C. Central nervous system disorders
      1. Encephalitis or meningitis, bacterial or viral
      2. Head trauma
      3. Brain abscess
      4. Guillain-Barré syndrome
      5. Subarachnoid hemorrhage or subdural hematoma
      6. Acute intermittent porphyria
      7. Peripheral neuropathy
      8. Psychosis
      9. Delirium tremens
     10. Cerebrovascular accident
     11. Cerebral atrophy
     12. Cavernous sinus thrombosis
     13. Hydrocephalus
     14. Rocky Mountain spotted fever
     15. Multiple sclerosis

  D. SIADH in endocrine disease
      1. Myxedema

  E. "Idiopathic" SIADH

III. Drugs
  A. Vasopressin
  B. Oxytocin
  C. Vincristine
  D. Chlorpropamide
  E. Thiazide diuretics
  F. Clofibrate
  G. Carbamazepine
  H. Nicotine
  I. Phenothiazines
  J. Cyclophosphamide
  K. Tricyclic antidepressants
  L. Haloperidol
  M. Monamine oxidase inhibitors

Adapted from: Robertson GL. In Felig P, Baxter JD, Broadus AE, Frohman LA, editors: *Endocrinology and metabolism*, ed 2. New York, 1987, McGraw-Hill, p. 369.

II-7 CAUSES OF HYPERTHYROIDISM

I. Graves' disease
II. Thyroiditis
  A. Subacute thyroiditis
  B. Painless thyroiditis
  C. Radiation thyroiditis
III. Exogenous hyperthyroidism
  A. Iatrogenic
  B. Factitious
  C. Iodine-induced
IV. Toxic multinodular goiter
V. Toxic uninodular goiter (thyroid adenoma)
VI. Ectopic hyperthyroidism (struma ovarii)
VII. Thyroid carcinoma
VIII. TSH excess
  A. Pituitary thyrotropin
  B. Trophoblastic tumors

Adapted from: Utiger RD, Frohman LA. In Felig P, Baxter JD, Broadus AE, Frohman LA, editors: *Endocrinology and metabolism*, ed 2. New York, 1987, McGraw-Hill, p. 418.

II-8 CLINICAL FEATURES OF HYPERTHYROIDISM

Symptoms	Physical signs	Diagnosis
Weight loss	Moist, warm, smooth skin	$\uparrow T_4$
Diarrhea	Tachycardia	$\uparrow$ Free T_4
Heat intolerance	Plummer's nails	$\uparrow T_3$
Nervousness	Ocular signs	$\uparrow$ RAI uptake
Excessive sweating	Exophthalmos	$\uparrow T_3$ resin
Emotional	Stare	uptake
instability	Lid lag	$\downarrow$ TSH (by
Polyphagia	Infrequent blinking	ultra-
Fatigue and	Difficulty with convergence	sensitive
weakness	Thyromegaly	method)
Palpitations	Thyroid bruit	
	Means-Lerman scratch/high pitched pulmonic sound	
	Atrial arrhythmias (especially atrial fibrillation)	
	Heart failure	
	Hepatomegaly	
	Abnormal liver tests	
	Pretibial myxedema	

II-9 CAUSES OF HYPOTHYROIDISM

- I. Thyroidal hypothyroidism
    - A. Insufficient functional tissue
        1. Thyroiditis*
        2. Following ^{131}I therapy or thyroidectomy
        3. Thyroid dysgenesis
        4. Infiltrations*
    - B. Defective biosynthesis of thyroid hormone
        1. Iodine deficiency*
        2. Congenital defects*
        3. Antithyroid agents*
        4. Iodine excess*
- II. Hypothyrotropic hypothyroidism
    - A. Pituitary hypothyroidism
    - B. Hypothalamic hypothyroidism
- III. Generalized resistance to thyroid hormones

*Hypothyroidism may be accompanied by goiter in these cases.

Adapted from: Utiger RD. In Felig P, Baxter JD, Broadus AE, Frohman LA, editors: *Endocrinology and metabolism*, ed 2. New York, 1987, McGraw-Hill, p. 445.

II-10 CLINICAL FEATURES OF HYPOTHYROIDISM

Symptoms	Signs	Diagnosis
Lethargy	Deep hoarse voice	↓ T_4
Constipation	Periorbital puffiness	↓ Free T_4
Cold intolerance	Pretibial myxedema	↓ T_3 resin uptake
Menorrhagia	Macroglossia	↑ TSH
Mental slowing	Decreased auditory acuity	↑ Cholesterol
Motor slowing	Pericardial effusion	↑ LDH
Anorexia	Cardiomegaly	↑ CPK
Weight gain	Ileus	↑ SGOT
Dry skin	Psychosis	
Dry brittle hair	Cerebellar ataxia	
Muscle aches	Prolonged relaxation phase of deep tendon reflexes	
	Stupor or coma	
	Bradycardia	
	Ascites	
	Loss of outer third of eyebrows	

II-11 CIRCUMSTANCES ASSOCIATED WITH ALTERED CONCENTRATION OF TBG

Increased TBG	Decreased TBG
Pregnancy	Androgenic and anabolic steroids
Newborn state	Large doses of glucocorticoid
Oral contraceptives and other sources of estrogen	Chronic liver disease
Tamoxifen	Severe systemic illness
Infectious and chronic active hepatitis	Active acromegaly
Biliary cirrhosis	Nephrosis
Acute intermittent porphyria	Genetically determined
Perphenazine	Asparaginase
Genetically determined	

Adapted from: Ingbar SH, Wartofsky L. In Braunwald E, Isselbacher KJ, Petersdorf RG, Wilson JD, Martin J, Fauci AS, Root RK, editors: *Harrison's principles of internal medicine*, ed 12. New York, 1991, McGraw-Hill, p. 1694.

II-12 THYROID TUMOR: HISTOLOGICAL CLASSIFICATION OF EPITHELIAL THYROID TUMORS ACCORDING TO THE WORLD HEALTH ORGANIZATION

I. Epithelial tumors
   A. Benign
      1. Follicular adenoma
      2. Others
   B. Malignant
      1. Follicular carcinoma
      2. Papillary carcinoma
      3. Squamous cell carcinoma
      4. Undifferentiated (anaplastic) carcinoma
         a. Spindle cell type
         b. Giant cell type
         c. Small cell type
      5. Medullary carcinoma
II. Nonepithelial tumors
   A. Benign
   B. Malignant
      1. Fibrosarcoma
      2. Others
III. Miscellaneous tumors
   A. Carcinosarcoma
   B. Malignant hemangioendothelioma
   C. Malignant lymphoma
   D. Teratomas
IV. Secondary tumors

Histological Typing of Thyroid Tumors, International Histologic Classification of Tumors, No. 11, Geneva, World Health Organization, 1974.

II-12 THYROID TUMOR: HISTOLOGICAL CLASSIFICATION OF EPITHELIAL THYROID TUMORS ACCORDING TO THE WORLD HEALTH ORGANIZATION (CONTINUED): CLINICAL STAGES OF THYROID CARCINOMA

Stage I	Intrathyroidal lesions only
Stage II	Nonfixed cervical metastases
Stage III	Fixed lymph node metastases or invasion into the neck outside the thyroid
Stage IV	Thyroid tumors with metastatic disease outside the neck

Modified from: Smedal ML and Salzman FA. *Am J Roentgenol* 99:352, 1967. Source adapted from: Burrow GN. In Felig P, Baxter JD, Broadus AE, Frohman LA, editors: *Endocrinology and metabolism*, ed 2. New York, 1987, McGraw-Hill, p. 495.

II-13 STATES ASSOCIATED WITH DE-CREASED PERIPHERAL CONVERSION OF T4 TO T3

I. Physiologic
   A. Fetal and early neonatal life
   B. Old age
II. Pathologic
   A. Fasting
   B. Malnutrition
   C. Systemic illness
   D. Physical trauma
   E. Postoperative state
   F. Drugs (propylthiouracil, dexamethasone, propranolol, amiodarone)
   G. Radiographic contrast agents (Oragrafin, Telepaque)

From: Ingbar SG, et al. In Braunwald E, Isselbacher KJ, Petersdorf RG, Wilson JD, Martin J, Fauci AS, Root RK, editors: *Harrison's principles of internal medicine*, ed 12. New York, 1991, McGraw-Hill, p. 1695

II-14 ADRENAL CORTICAL INSUFFICIENCY

I. Etiology of primary adrenocortical insufficiency
  A. Idiopathic/autoimmune (≅80%)
  B. Tuberculosis (≅20%)
  C. Miscellaneous (≅1%)
    1. (1) Hemorrhage: sepsis, anticoagulants, coagulopathy, trauma, surgery, pregnancy, neonatal
       (2) Infarction: thrombosis, embolism, arteritis
    2. Fungal infection: histoplasmosis, coccidioidomycosis, blastomycosis, moniliasis, torulosis
    3. Metastatic neoplasm
    4. Lymphoma
    5. Amyloidosis
    6. Sarcoidosis
    7. Hemochromatosis
    8. Surgery: bilateral adrenalectomy
    9. Enzyme inhibitors: metyrapone, aminoglutethimide, trilostane
    10. Cytotoxic agents: o,p´-DDD
    11. Congenital: adrenal hyperplasia, hypoplasia, familial glucocorticoid deficiency
    12. Acquired immunodeficiency syndrome
    13. Irradiation

II. Clinical disorders associated with idiopathic adrenocortical insufficiency

A. Primary ovarian failure		23%
B. Thyroid		
	1. Thyrotoxicosis	7%
	2. Hypothyroidism/chronic thyroiditis	9%
C. Diabetes mellitus		12%
D. Vitiligo		9%
E. Hypoparathyroidism		6%
F. Pernicious anemia		4%

Modified from: Irvine WJ, Barnes EW. Adrenocortical insufficiency. *Clin Endocrinol Metab* 1:549-594, 1972. Adapted from: Baxter JD, et al. In Felig P, Baxter JD, Broadus AE, Frohman LA, editors: *Endocrinology and metabolism,* ed 2. New York, 1987, McGraw-Hill, p. 582.

II-15 CLINICAL FEATURES OF ADDISON'S DISEASE

Symptoms and physical signs	Diagnosis
I. Anorexia	I. ↓ plasma cortisol
II. Weakness and easy fatigability	A. Little increase after synthetic ACTH
III. Nausea and vomiting	B. ↑ ACTH levels with primary adrenal failure
IV. Weight loss	II. ↓ urinary 17-hydroxy and 17-ketosteroid
V. Salt craving	III. Hyponatremia
VI. Diarrhea	IV. Hyperkalemia
VII. Postural hypotension	V. Anemia
VIII. Hyperpigmentation	VI. Eosinophilia
IX. Personality changes	VII. Reduction in heart size
X. Decrease in axillary and pubic hair	VIII. Hypercalcemia (rare)
XI. Muscle and joint pains	
XII. Amenorrhea	

II-16 CUSHING'S SYNDROME

I. Classification and etiology
  A. ACTH dependent:
    1. Cushing's disease — 68%
    2. Ectopic ACTH syndrome — 15%
  B. ACTH independent:
    1. Adrenal adenoma — 9%
    2. Adrenal carcinoma — 8%
                 100%

Reference: Huff TA. Clinical syndromes related to disorders of adreno-corticotrophic hormone. In Allen MB, Makesh VB, editors: *The pituitary: a current review.* New York, 1977, Academic Press, pp. 153-168.

II. Tumors most frequently causing the ectopic ACTH syndrome
  A. Oat cell carcinoma of the lung
  B. Thymoma
  C. Pancreatic islet cell carcinoma
  D. Carcinoid tumors (lung, gut, pancreas, ovary)
  E. Thyroid medullary carcinoma
  F. Pheochromocytoma and related tumors

Adapted from: Baxter JD, et al. In Felig P, Baxter JD, Broadus AE, Frohman LA, editors: *Endocrinology and metabolism,* ed 2. New York, 1987, McGraw-Hill, p. 604.

II-17 CLINICAL FEATURES OF CUSHING'S SYNDROME

Clinical features	Diagnosis
I. Typical facial feature and habitus	I. Plasma cortisol usually ↑ No suppression with pm dexamethasone
II. Weight gain	
III. Weakness and easy fatigability	
IV. Amenorrhea	II. ↑ urinary 17-hydroxy-corticoid; ↑ free cortisol
V. Personality changes	
VI. Polyuria, polydipsia	III. Suppression of plasma cortisol and urinary hydroxycorticoids by low or high dose dexamethasone
VII. Hypertension	
VIII. Hirsutism, striae, ecchymosis	
IX. Edema	
X. Clitoral hypertrophy	
	IV. Mild leukocytosis
	V. Eosinopenia
	VI. Hypokalemic acidosis
	VII. Hyperglycemia
	VIII. CT scan may be of value

II-18 SYNDROME OF PRIMARY ALDOSTERONISM

I. Etiology
   A. Aldosterone-producing adenoma
   B. Adrenocortical hyperplasia
      1. Idiopathic aldosteronism (aldosterone production-nonsuppressible)
      2. Indeterminate aldosteronism (aldosterone production-suppressible)
      3. Glucocorticoid-suppressible aldosteronism
      4. Surgically remediable aldosteronism (?)
   C. Adrenocortical carcinoma
II. Clinical features
   A. Symptoms and signs
      1. Hypertension
      2. Muscle weakness
      3. Polyuria
      4. Polydipsia
   B. Diagnosis
      1. Hypokalemia
      2. Hypernatremia (occasional)
      3. Alkaline to neutral urine pH
      4. Metabolic alkalosis
      5. Hyperglycemia
      6. Failure of plasma renin to rise normally
         a. Diuretics
         b. Upright
         c. Sodium depletion
      7. CT scan may be helpful

II-19 CLASSIFICATION OF SECONDARY HYPERALDOSTERONISM

Primary abnormality	Potassium loss	Edema	Hypertension	Effect of sodium load
Extrarenal sodium loss Hemorrhage Thermal stress Gastrointestinal loss	Absent	Absent	Absent	Repairs deficit
Sodium restriction	Absent	Absent	Absent	Repairs deficit
Abnormal distribution of sodium excess Congestive heart failure Nephrotic syndrome Cirrhosis with ascites Idiopathic edema	Present	Present	Absent	Worsens edema
Abnormal renal electrolyte loss Salt-losing renal disease Bartter's syndrome Diuretic abuse Renal tubular acidosis	Present	Absent	Absent	Variable

II-19 CLASSIFICATION OF SECONDARY HYPERALDOSTERONISM (CONTINUED)

Primary abnormality	Potassium loss	Edema	Hypertension	Effect of sodium load
Other renal lesions Renal artery stenosis* Unilateral renal ischemia Accelerated hypertension Renin-secreting tumor Chronic renal failure*	Present	Absent	Present	May worsen hypertension
Excessive potassium intake	Present	Absent	Absent	May facilitate kaluresis
Luteal phase of menstrual cycle and pregnancy	Absent	May be Present	Usually Present	Suppresses renin and aldosterone

*Exception; no potassium loss

Modified from Stockigt JR. Mineralocorticoid excess. In James VHT, editor: *The Adrenal Gland.* New York, 1979, Raven Press, pp. 197-242.
Adapted from: Baxter JD, et al. In Felig P, Baxter JD, Broadus AE, Frohman LA, editors: *Endocrinology and metabolism*, ed 2. New York, 1987, McGraw-Hill, p. 621.

II-20 CAUSES OF HYPOMAGNESEMIA AND MAGNESIUM DEPLETION

I. Decreased intake and/or absorption
   A. Protein-calorie malnutrition
   B. Losses of gastrointestinal fluids
   C. Malabsorption
   D. Primary hypomagnesemia
   E. Parenteral hyperalimentation without adequate magnesium

II. Renal losses
   A. Osmotic diuresis; mannitol, glucose, urea
   B. Following relief of obstruction or renal tubular acidosis
   C. Post-renal transplant
   D. Drugs: Loop diuretics, cisplatin, entamicin, amphotericin, digoxin, capreomycin, viomycin, tobramycin, amikacin
   E. ECF expansion, Bartter's syndrome, hyperaldosteronism
   F. Congenital, hereditary wasting

III. Miscellaneous disorders
   A. Chronic alcoholism
   B. Diabetic ketoacidosis/diabetes mellitus
   C. Primary hyperparathyroidism
   D. Post-parathyroidectomy
   E. Chronic hypoparathyroidism
   F. Hyperthyroidism
   G. SIADH
   H. Hypoalbuminemia
   I. Dialysis
   J. Excessive lactation
   K. Pancreatitis

Adapted from: Stewart AF, Broadus AE, Frohman LA. In Felig P, Baxter JD, Broadus AE, Frohman LA, editors: *Endocrinology and metabolism*, ed 2. New York, 1987, McGraw-Hill, p. 1439.

II-21 CLASSIFICATION OF DIABETES MELLITUS

I. Spontaneous diabetes mellitus
   A. Type I or insulin-dependent diabetes (formerly called juvenile-onset diabetes)
   B. Type II or insulin-independent diabetes (formerly called maturity-onset diabetes)
II. Secondary diabetes
   A. Pancreatic disease (pancreoprival diabetes, e.g., pancreatectomy, pancreatic insufficiency, hemochromatosis)
   B. Hormonal: excess secretion of counterregulatory hormones (e.g., acromegaly, Cushing's syndrome, pheochromocytoma)
   C. Drug induced (e.g., potassium-losing diuretics, contrainsulin hormones, psychoactive agents, diphenylhydantoin)
   D. Associated with complex genetic syndrome (e.g., ataxia telangiectasia, Laurence-Moon-Biedl syndrome, myotonic dystrophy, Friedreich's ataxia)
III. Impaired glucose tolerance (formerly called chemical diabetes, asymptomatic diabetes, latent diabetes, and subclinical diabetes): Normal fasting plasma glucose, and 2-h value on glucose tolerance test > 140 mg/dL but < 200 mg/dL
IV. Gestational diabetes: glucose intolerance which has its onset in pregnancy

Sources: National Diabetes Data Group: *Diabetes* 28:1039, 1979. Adapted from Shatrir E, Bergman M. In Felig P, Baxter JD, Broadus AE, Frohman LA, editors: *Endocrinology and metabolism,* ed 2. New York, 1987, McGraw-Hill, p. 1093.

II-22 PRECIPITATING FACTORS IN DIABETIC KETOACIDOSIS

I. Infection
   A. Urinary tract
   B. Pneumonias
   C. Cellulitis
   D. Periodontal
   E. Central nervous system
   F. Septicemia
II. Metabolic/endocrine
   A. Uremia
   B. Hypothyroidism
   C. Cushing's syndrome
III. Dietary indiscretion
IV. Not taking insulin
V. Pregnancy
VI. Myocardial infarction
VII. CVA
VIII. Drugs
   A. Thiazides
   B. Corticosteroids
IX. Acute pancreatitis
X. Excessive alcohol consumption

II-23 MAJOR CAUSES OF FASTING HYPOGLYCEMIA

I. Conditions primarily due to underproduction of glucose
  A. Hormone deficiencies
    1. Hypopituitarism
    2. Adrenal insufficiency
    3. Catecholamine deficiency
    4. Glucagon deficiency
  B. Enzyme defects
    1. Glucose 6-phosphatase
    2. Liver phosphorylase
    3. Pyruvate carboxylase
    4. Phosphoenolpyruvate carboxykinase
    5. Fructose 1,6-diphosphatase
    6. Glycogen synthetase
  C. Substrate deficiency
    1. Ketotic hypoglycemia of infancy
    2. Severe malnutrition, muscle wasting
    3. Late pregnancy
  D. Acquired liver disease
    1. Hepatic congestion
    2. Severe hepatitis
    3. Cirrhosis
    4. Uremia
    5. Hypothermia
  E. Drugs
    1. Alcohol
    2. Propranolol
    3. Salicylates
II. Conditions primarily due to overutilization of glucose
  A. Hyperinsulinism
    1. Insulinoma
    2. Exogenous insulin
    3. Sulfonylureas
    4. Deficiency in enzymes of fat oxidation
    5. 3-Hydroxy-3-methylglutaryl-CoA lyase deficiency
  B. Appropriate insulin levels
    1. Extrapancreatic tumors
    2. Carnitine deficiency
    3. Cachexia with fat depletion
    4. Deficiency in enzymes of fat oxidation

Adapted from: Foster DW, Rubenstein AH. In Braunwald E, Isselbacher KJ, Petersdorf RG, Wilson JD, Martin J, Fauci AS, Root RK, editors: *Harrison's principles of internal medicine*, ed 12. New York, 1991, McGraw-Hill, p. 1761.

II-24 INSULIN RESISTANT STATES

   I. Prereceptor resistance
      A. Mutated insulins
      B. Anti-insulin antibodies
  II. Receptor and postreceptor resistance
      A. Obesity
      B. Type A syndrome (absent or dysfunctional receptor)
      C. Type B syndrome (antibody to insulin receptor)
      D. Lipodystrophic states (partial or generalized)
      E. Leprechaunism
      F. Ataxia — telangiectasia
      G. Rabson-Mendenhall syndrome
      H. Werner syndrome
      I. Alström's syndrome
      J. Pineal hyperplasia syndrome

Adapted from: Foster DW. In Braunwald E, Isselbacher KJ, Petersdorf RG, Wilson JD, Martin J, Fauci AS, Root RK, editors: *Harrison's principles of internal medicine*, ed 12. New York, 1991, McGraw-Hill, p. 1757.

II-25 A CLASSIFICATION OF THE OBESITIES

I. Etiologic
  A. Hypothalamic dysfunction
    1. Tumors
    2. Inflammation
    3. Trauma and surgical injury
    4. Increased intracranial pressure
    5. Functional changes causing hyperinsulinemia?
  B. Endocrine
    1. Glucocorticoid excess (Cushing's syndrome)
    2. Thyroid hormone deficiency (hypothyroidism)
    3. Hypopituitarism
    4. Gonadal deficiency (primary and secondary hypogonadism)
    5. Hyperinsulinism (insulinoma, excess exogenous insulin)
  C. Genetic
    1. Inherited predisposition to obesity
    2. Genetic syndromes associated with obesity:
      a. Prader-Willi syndrome
      b. Alström's syndrome
      c. Laurence-Moon-Bardet-Biedl syndrome
      d. Stewart-Morel-Morgagni syndrome (hyperostosis frontalis internal)
      e. Down's syndrome
      f. Pseudo- and pseudo-pseudo-hypoparathyroidism
  D. Nutritional
    1. Maternal nutritional factors?
    2. Infant feeding practices?
    3. Excess caloric intake during adulthood
  E. Drugs
    1. Phenothiazines
    2. Insulin
    3. Corticosteroids
    4. Cyproheptadine
    5. Tricyclic antidepressants
II. Anatomic
  A. Hypercellular-hypertrophic: early age of onset, severe obesity
  B. Hypertrophic-normal cellular; adult onset, milder obesity
III. Contributory factors
  A. Familial influences
  B. Physical inactivity
  C. Dietary factors: eating patterns, type of diet
  D. Socioeconomic
  E. Educational
  F. Cultural-ethnic
  G. Psychologic

II-25 A CLASSIFICATION OF THE OBESITIES (CONTINUED)

Adapted from: Salans LB. In Felig P, Baxter JD, Broadus AE, Frohman LA, editors: *Endocrinology and metabolism*, ed 2. New York, 1987, McGraw-Hill, p. 1225.

II-26 HYPERCALCEMIC CONDITIONS ARRANGED BY CATEGORY IN DESCENDING ORDER OF APPROXIMATE FREQUENCY

I. Primary hyperparathyroidism
  A. Sporadic
  B. Clinical variants and familial syndromes
II. Neoplastic diseases
  A. Local osteolysis
  B. Humoral hypercalcemia of malignancy (PTH)
  C. Lymphoma-associated hypercalcemia
III. Endocrinopathies
  A. Thyrotoxicosis
  B. Adrenal insufficiency
  C. Pheochromocytoma
  D. VIP-oma syndrome
IV. Medications
  A. Thiazide diuretics
  B. Vitamins A and D
  C. Milk alkali syndrome
  D. Lithium
  E. Estrogens and anti-estrogens
V. Sarcoidosis and other granulomatous diseases
VI. Miscellaneous conditions
  A. Immobilization
  B. Acute renal failure
  C. Idiopathic hypercalcemia of infancy
  D. Serum protein abnormalities

Adapted from: Stewart AF, Broadus AE. In Felig P, Baxter JD, Broadus AE, Frohman LA, editors: *Endocrinology and metabolism*, ed 2. New York, 1987, McGraw-Hill, p. 1422.

II-27 HYPOPARATHYROIDISM

    I. Postoperative hypocalcemia and hypoparathyroidism
   II. Idiopathic hypoparathyroidism
      A. Isolated
      B. Associated with atrophic polyendocrine failure
  III. Other acquired forms of functional hypoparathyroidism
      A. Nonsurgical parathyroid damage
      B. Parathyroid infiltration
      C. Hypomagnesemia
  IV. Pseudohypoparathyroidism
   V. Neonatal hypocalcemic syndromes
      A. Early and late neonatal hypocalcemia
      B. Secondary hypoparathyroidism
      C. DiGeorge's syndrome and idiopathic hypoparathyroidism

Adapted from: Stewart AF, Broadus AE. In Felig P, Baxter JD, Broadus AE, Frohman LA, editors: *Endocrinology and metabolism,* ed 2. New York, 1987, McGraw-Hill, p. 1422.

II-28 NONHYPOPARATHYROID HYPOCALCEMIA CONDITIONS

    I. Renal insufficiency
      A. Reduced $1,25\text{-}(OH)_2D$
      B. Hypophosphatemic
   II. Vitamin D deficiency, rickets, and osteomalacia
      A. Simple vitamin D deficiency
      B. Intestinal malabsorption
      C. Hepatic and biliary disorders
      D. Anticonvulsant therapy
      E. Vitamin D-dependent rickets
      F. Vitamin D-resistant (hypophosphatemic) rickets and osteomalacia
  III. Acute pancreatitis
  IV. Rapid or excessive skeletal mineralization
      A. Hungry bones syndrome
      B. Osteoblastic metastases
      C. Vitamin D therapy for vitamin D disorders
   V. Hypoalbuminemia
  VI. Hypophosphatemia
      A. Parenteral phosphorus
      B. Phosphate-containing enemas
      C. Excessive oral phosphorus
      D. Renal failure
      E. Crush injuries
      F. Rapid tumor lysis

II-28 NONHYPOPARATHYROID HYPOCALCEMIA CONDITIONS (CONTINUED)

   VII. Hypomagnesemia
  VIII. Toxic shock syndrome
    IX. Medications
       A. Plicamyacin (formerly mithramycin)
       B. Citrated blood
       C. Fluoride intoxication
       D. Calcitonin

Adapted from: Stewart AF, Broadus AE, Frohman LA. In Felig P, Baxter JD, Broadus AE, Frohman LA, editors: *Endocrinology and metabolism*, ed 2. New York, 1987, McGraw-Hill, p. 1422.

II-29 CLASSIFICATION OF OSTEOMALACIA AND RICKETS

    I. Reduction of circulating vitamin D metabolites
       A. Inadequate ultraviolet light exposure and inadequate dietary vitamin D
       B. Vitamin D malabsorption
         1. Small intestinal disease
         2. Pancreatic insufficiency
         3. Insufficient bile salts
       C. Abnormal vitamin D metabolism
         1. Liver disease
         2. Chronic renal failure
         3. Drugs (anticonvulsants, glutethimide)
         4. Mesenchymal tumors, prostatic cancer
         5. Vitamin D-dependent rickets type I (25-hydroxyvitamin D 1α-hydroxylase deficiency)
       D. Renal loss
         1. Nephrotic syndrome
    II. Peripheral resistance to vitamin D
       A. Vitamin D-dependent rickets, type II
       B. Anticonvulsant drugs
       C. Chronic renal failure
   III. Hypophosphatemia
       A. Renal phosphate wasting
         1. Hypophosphatemic wasting
           a. Familial X-linked
           b. Autosomal recessive
           c. Sporadic

II-29 CLASSIFICATION OF OSTEOMALACIA AND RICKETS (CONTINUED)

    2. Hypophosphatemic osteomalacia
      a. Familial X-linked
      b. Sporadic
    3. Fanconi syndrome
    4. Mesenchymal tumors, fibrous dysplasias, epidermal nevus syndrome, prostatic cancer
    5. Primary hyperparathyroidism
    6. Familial renal phosphate leak with hypercalciuria, nephrolithiasis and osteomalacia and rickets
  B. Malnutrition
  C. Malabsorption due to gastrointestinal disease or phosphate-binding antacids
  D. Chronic dialysis
IV. Miscellaneous
  A. Inhibitors of calcification
    1. Sodium fluoride
    2. Disodium etidronate
  B. Calcium deficiency
  C. Hypophosphatasia
  D. Fibrogenesis imperfecta ossium
  E. Hypoparathyroidism
  F. Systemic acidosis
  G. Total parenteral nutrition

Adapted from: Singer FR, Frohman LA. In Felig P, Baxter JD, Broadus AE, Frohman LA, editors: *Endocrinology and metabolism,* ed 2. New York, 1987, McGraw-Hill, p. 1462.

II-30 CLASSIFICATION OF OSTEOPOROSIS

   I. Aging
   II. Endocrine abnormality
      A. Estrogen deficiency
      B. Testosterone deficiency
      C. Cushing's syndrome
      D. Thyrotoxicosis
      E. Primary hyperparathyroidism
      F. Diabetes mellitus
   III. Nutritional abnormality
      A. Vitamin C deficiency
      B. Protein deficiency
   IV. Immobilization or weightlessness
   V. Hematologic malignancy
      A. Multiple myeloma
      B. Leukemia
      C. Lymphoma
   VI. Genetic
      A. Osteogenesis imperfecta
      B. Ehlers-Danlos syndrome
      C. Homocystinuria
      D. Marfan's syndrome
      E. Menkes' syndrome
   VII. Systemic mastocytosis
   VIII. Heparin therapy
   IX. Rheumatoid arthritis
   X. Chronic liver disease
   XI. Juvenile osteoporosis
   XII. Idiopathic
   XIII. Chronic hypophosphatemia
   XIV. Chronic alcoholism

Adapted from: Singer FR, Frohman LA. In Felig P, Baxter JD, Broadus AE, Frohman LA, editors: *Endocrinology and metabolism*, ed 2. New York, 1987, McGraw-Hill, p. 1471.

II-31 CLINICAL RISK FACTORS FOR CALCIUM STONE FORMATION

I. General issues and/or risk factors
   A. Positive family history
   B. Medications (vitamins A, D, C, absorbable antacids, acetazolamide)
   C. Urinary pH
   D. Diet
II. Specific, treatable risk factors
   A. Low urine volume
   B. Hypercalciuria
   C. Hyperoxaluria
   D. Hyperuricosuria
   E. Hypocitraturia

Adapted from: Singer FR, Frohman LA. In Felig P, Baxter JD, Broadus AE, Frohman LA, editors: *Endocrinology and metabolism*, ed 2. New York, 1987, McGraw-Hill, p. 1529.

II-32 CAUSES OF HIRSUTISM IN FEMALES

I. Familial
II. Idiopathic
III. Ovarian
   A. Polycystic ovaries; hilus-cell hyperplasia
   B. Tumor; arrhenoblastoma, hilus cell, adrenal rest
IV. Adrenal
   A. Congenital adrenal hyperplasia
   B. Noncongenital adrenal hyperplasia (Cushing's)
   C. Tumor; virilizing carcinoma or adenoma
V. Drugs: minoxidil, androgens

Adapted from: Williams GW, Dluhy RG. In Braunwald E, Isselbacher KJ, Petersdorf RG, Wilson JD, Martin J, Fauci AS, Root RK, editors: *Harrison's principles of internal medicine*, ed 12. New York, 1991, McGraw-Hill, p. 1728.

II-33 CAUSES OF AMENORRHEA

I. Primary Amenorrhea
  A. Gonadal dysgenesis (Turner's syndrome)
  B. Pure gonadal dysgenesis (XX gonadal dysgenesis)
  C. Swyer's syndrome (XY gonadal dysgenesis)
  D. Testicular feminization
  E. Pelvic anatomic abnormalities
    1. Uterine agenesis
    2. Cervical stenosis
    3. Intrauterine synechiae
    4. Imperforate hymen
  F. Hypothalamic and pituitary tumors
    1. Craniopharyngioma
    2. Dysgerminoma
    3. Prolactin secreting tumors
  G. Systemic Illness
  H. Weight loss
  I. Stress
  J. Athletic training
  K. "Physiologic delay" of puberty
  L. Hypogonadotropic hypogonadism (Kallmann's syndrome)
II. Secondary Amenorrhea
  A. Premature menopause
  B. Autoimmune ovarian failure
  C. "Resistant" ovary syndrome
  D. Stress, weight loss, exercise
  E. Systemic disease
  F. Prolactin secreting pituitary microadenoma
  G. Destructive or infiltrative hypothalamic or pituitary lesions
  H. Virilizing syndromes
    1. Idiopathic hirsutism
    2. Polycystic ovarian disease
    3. Attenuated forms of congenital adrenal hyperplasia
    4. Insulin resistance
    5. Loss of endometrium (Asherman's syndrome)

Adapted from: *Endocrinology and metabolism,* MKSAP VII, American College of Physicians, pp. 220-221, 1986.

II-34 DIFFERENTIAL DIAGNOSIS OF GYNECOMASTIA

I. Physiological gynecomastia
   A. Newborn
   B. Adolescence
   C. Aging
II. Pathological gynecomastia
   A. Deficient production or action of testosterone
      1. Congenital anorchia
      2. Klinefelter's syndrome
      3. Androgen resistance (testicular feminization and Reifenstein's syndrome)
      4. Defects in testosterone synthesis
      5. Secondary testicular failure (viral orchitis, trauma castration, neurological and granulomatous diseases, renal failure)
   B. Increased estrogen production
      1. Estrogen secretion
         a. True hermaphroditism
         b. Testicular tumors
         c. Carcinoma of the lung and other tumors producing HCG
      2. Increased substrate for peripheral aromatase
         a. Adrenal disease
         b. Liver disease
         c. Starvation
         d. Thyrotoxicosis
      3. Increase in peripheral aromatase
   C. Drugs
      1. Inhibitors of testosterone synthesis and/or action (spironolactone, cimetidine, alkylating agents, cisplatin, metronidazole, ketoconazole, finesteride).
      2. Estrogens (diethylstilbestrol, birth control pills, digitalis, estrogen containing cosmetics or foods).
      3. Drugs that enhance endogenous estrogen secretion (clomiphene, gonadotropins)
      4. Unknown mechanisms (busulfan, isoniazid, methyldopa, tricyclic antidepressants, D-penicillamine, diazepam, marijuana, heroin)
   D. Idiopathic

Adapted from: Wilson JD. In Braunwald E, Isselbacher KJ, Petersdorf RG, Wilson JD, Martin J, Fauci AS, Root RK, editors: *Harrison's principles of internal medicine*, ed 12. New York, 1991, McGraw-Hill, p. 1797.

II-35 CLASSIFICATION OF HYPERLIPIDEMIAS BASED ON LIPOPROTEIN CONCENTRATIONS

Type	Lipoprotein abnormality	Lipid profiles	Typical values mg/dl
I	Chylomicrons markedly ↑ VLDL and LDL both normal or low	Chol ↑ Tg ↑↑	320 4000
IIa	LDL ↑, VLDL normal	Chol ↑ Tg N	370 90
IIb	LDL ↑, VLDL ↑	Chol ↑ Tg ↑	350 400
III	Abnormal cholesterol-enriched VLDL present in excess	Chol ↑ Tg ↑	500 700
IV	VLDL ↑, LDL normal	Chol N Tg ↑	220
V	Chylomicrons markedly ↑, VLDL ↑, LDL normal or low	Chol ↑ Tg ↑↑	700 5000

Source: Based on Fredrickson, Levy, and Lees and the WHO Committee

II-36 RELATIVE ATHEROGENICITY OF INDIVIDUAL LIPOPROTEIN PARTICLES

Lipoprotein	Atherogenicity	Typical associated dyslipoproteinemia
Chylomicrons (lipoprotein lipase deficiency)	0	Type I
VLDL	+	Type IV (familial hypertriglyceridemia)
Chylomicron and VLDL remnants	+++	Type III (dysbeta-lipoproteinemia)
LDL	++++	Type II (familial hypercholesterolemia)
HDL	Negatively correlated with atherosclerosis	Familial hyperalphalipoproteinemia

Adapted from: Illingworth R, Connor WE. In Felig P, Baxter JD, Broadus AE, Frohman LA, editors: *Endocrinology and metabolism*, ed 2. New York, 1987, McGraw-Hill, p. 1255-F.

II-37 PRIMARY VERSUS SECONDARY HYPERLIPIDEMIAS

I. Primary: genetic
II. Secondary:
   A. Diet: excessive cholesterol, saturated fat, or calories
   B. Uncontrolled diabetes
   C. Alcohol
   D. Hypothyroidism
   E. Nephrotic syndrome
   F. Chronic renal failure
   G. Biliary obstruction; primary biliary cirrhosis
   H. Dysglobulinemia; autoimmune disease
   I. Glycogen storage disease
   J. Acute intermittent porphyria
   K. Cushing's syndrome
   L. Anorexia nervosa
   M. Hepatoma
   N. Drug-induced: corticosteroids, estrogens, thiazides, beta blockers, 13-*cis*-retinoic acid (isotretinoin [Accutane])

Adapted from: Illingworth R, Connor WE. In Felig P, Baxter JD, Broadus AE, Frohman LA, editors: *Endocrinology and metabolism,* ed 2. New York, 1987, McGraw-Hill, p. 1255-F.

II-38 SOME ORGANIC CAUSES OF ERECTILE IMPOTENCE IN MEN

I. Neurological diseases
   A. Anterior temporal lobe lesions
   B. Diseases of the spinal cord
   C. Loss of sensory input
      1. Tabes dorsalis
      2. Disease of dorsal root ganglia
   D. Disease of nervi erigentes
      1. Complete prostatectomy
      2. Rectosigmoid operations
   E. Diabetic autonomic neuropathy and various polyneuropathies
II. Endocrine causes
   A. Testicular failure (primary or secondary)
   B. Hyperprolactinemia
III. Drugs
   A. Antihistamines
      1. Cimetidine
      2. Diphenhydramine
      3. Hydroxyzine

II-38 SOME ORGANIC CAUSES OF ERECTILE IMPOTENCE IN MEN (CONTINUED)

   B. Antihypertensives
      1. Clonidine
      2. Methyldopa
      3. Propranolol
      4. Reserpine
      5. Spironolactone
      6. Thiazides
   C. Anticholinergics
   D. Antidepressants
      1. Amitriptyline
      2. Doxepin
      3. Isocarboxazid
   E. Antipsychotics
      1. Chlorpromazine
      2. Haloperidol
      3. Thioridazine
   F. Tranquilizers
      1. Diazepam
      2. Barbiturates
      3. Chlordiazepoxide
   G. Drugs of habituation or addiction
      1. Alcohol
      2. Methadone
      3. Heroin
IV. Vascular diseases: Leriche's syndrome
 V. Penile diseases
   A. Previous priapism
   B. Penile trauma
   C. Peyronie's disease

Modified from: Wilson JD, McConnell JD, et al. In Braunwald E, Isselbacher KJ, Petersdorf RG, Wilson JD, Martin J, Fauci AS, Root RK, editors: *Harrison's principles of internal medicine*, ed 12. New York, 1991, McGraw-Hill, p. 297.

II-39 HYPOPHOSPHATEMIA

   I. Increased excretion of phosphorus in the urine
     A. Primary hyperparathyroidism
     B. Secondary hyperparathyroidism
     C. Renal tubular defects
     D. Diuretic phase of acute tubular necrosis
     E. Postobstructive diuresis
     F. Postrenal transplantation
     G. ECF volume expansion
   II. Abnormalities of vitamin D metabolism
     A. Vitamin D-deficient rickets
     B. Familial hypophosphatemic rickets
     C. Vitamin D-dependent rickets
     D. Hypophosphatemia associated with tumors
   III. Decrease in gastrointestinal absorption of phosphorus
     A. Malabsorption
     B. Malnutrition-starvation
     C. Administration of phosphate binders
   IV. Miscellaneous causes
     A. Diabetes mellitus: during treatment for ketoacidosis
     B. Severe respiratory alkalosis
     C. Recovery phase of malnutrition
     D. Alcohol withdrawal
     E. Toxic shock syndrome
     F. Leukemia, lymphoma
     G. Severe burns

Reference: Slatopolsky E, Klahr S. In Schrier RW, Gottschalk MD, editors: *Diseases of the Kidney*, ed 5. Boston, 1993, Little, Brown, p. 2604.

II-40 COMPLICATIONS OF CORTICOSTEROID THERAPY

   I. Stigmata of hypercorticism
     A. Acne
     B. Hirsutism
     C. Moon facies
     D. Cervico-thoracic obesity
     E. Striae
     F. Easy bruisability
     G. Impaired wound healing
   II. Problems secondary to abnormalities of salt and water metabolism
     A. Sodium retention
     B. Weight gain (also increased appetite and polyphagia)

II-40 COMPLICATIONS OF CORTICOSTEROID THERAPY (CONTINUED)

  - C. Edema
  - D. Increased blood pressure
  - E. Hypokalemia (muscle weakness)
- III. Endocrine-metabolic problems
  - A. Unmask latent diabetes
  - B. Aggravate manifest diabetes
  - C. Potential for adrenal crises with abrupt discontinuation of Rx or stress
- IV. Musculoskeletal
  - A. Steroid myopathy with muscle weakness
  - B. Osteopenia
  - C. Compression fractures
  - D. Aseptic necrosis of femoral head
- V. Gastrointestinal
  - A. Vague abdominal pain
  - B. Dyspepsia
  - C. ? — likelihood of peptic ulcer
  - D. ? — likelihood of GI bleeding
  - E. Pancreatitis
  - F. Mask an acute abdomen
- VI. Psychiatric
  - A. Depression
  - B. Euphoria
  - C. Insomnia
  - D. Irritability
  - E. Psychosis
- VII. Hematologic
  - A. Leukocytosis
  - B. Neutrophilia
  - C. Lymphocytopenia
- VIII. Immunologic-infectious
  - A. False negative skin tests
  - B. Increased susceptibility to infections
  - C. Opportunistic infections
  - D. Reactivation of tuberculosis
  - E. Impaired cell mediated immunity
- IX. Miscellaneous
  - A. Premature cataracts

II-41 SOME CAUSES OF HYPERLACTATEMIA

I. Hyperlactatemia with hypoxia
  A. Strenuous muscle exercise (convulsions, hypothermia)
  B. Inadequate tissue perfusion or oxygenation of any cause*
II. Hyperlactatemia without apparent hypoxia
  A. Systemic clinical disorders
    1. Alkalosis (respiratory or metabolic)
    2. Uncontrolled diabetes mellitus
    3. Leukemia, lymphoma, other cancers
    4. Severe liver disease
    5. Thiamine deficiency
  B. Drugs, hormones, toxins
    1. Phenformin and other biguanides
    2. Salicylates
    3. Sodium nitroprusside
    4. Ethanol
    5. Epinephrine, glucagon
    6. Fructose, sorbitol
  C. Enzyme defects
    1. Glucose 6-phosphatase
    2. Fructose 1,6-bisphosphatase
    3. Pyruvate carboxylase
    4. Pyruvate dehydrogenase
    5. Unclassified tricarboxylic acid defect
  D. Certain primary myopathies
  E. Idiopathic

*The most common causes of perfusion-oxygenation defects are myocardial infarction, sepsis, hemorrhage, volume depletion, pulmonary embolism, and heart failure. Hypoxia due to severe pulmonary disease, chronic anemia, carbon monoxide inhalation, and cyanide poisoning are much less frequent.

Source: After Cohen and Woods, 1976.

Adapted from: Foster DW. In Braunwald E, Isselbacher KJ, Petersdorf RG, Wilson JD, Martin J, Fauci AS, Root RK, editors: *Harrison's principles of internal medicine*, ed 12. New York, 1991, McGraw-Hill, p. 1799.

II-42 LATE COMPLICATIONS OF DIABETES MELLITUS

   I. Atherosclerosis
      A. Coronary artery disease
      B. Cerebrovascular disease
      C. Peripheral vascular disease
   II. Retinopathy
      A. Background
      B. Proliferative
  III. Neuropathy
      A. Peripheral polyneuropathy
      B. Mononeuropathy
      C. Radiculopathy
      D. Amyotrophy
      E. Autonomic neuropathy with esophageal dysfunction, delayed gastric emptying, diarrhea, constipation, neurogenic bladder, impotence and orthostatic hypotension.
  IV. Nephropathy
   V. Cardiomyopathy
  VI. Hypertriglyceridemia
 VII. Hyporeninemic hypoaldosteronism
VIII. Skin and soft tissue problems
      A. Necrobiosis lipoidica diabeticorum
      B. Diabetic dermopathy
      C. Adipose atrophy or hypertrophy
      D. Impaired wound healing
      E. Foot ulcers
  IX. Increased susceptibility to infections
   X. Cataracts
  XI. Nonalcoholic steatohepatitis

CHAPTER III
GASTROENTEROLOGY

III-1 CLASSIFICATION OF ESOPHAGEAL MOTILITY DISORDERS

I. Primary
   A. Achalasia
   B. Diffuse esophageal spasm
   C. Variants of achalasia and diffuse esophageal spasm
II. Secondary
   A. Collagen disease
      1. Scleroderma
      2. Systemic lupus erythematosus
      3. Raynaud's disease
      4. Dermatomyositis, polymyositis
   B. Physical, chemical and pharmacologic
      1. Vagotomy
      2. Radiation
      3. Chemical: reflux esophagitis
      4. Drugs (atropine, belladonna alkaloids, Ca^{++} channel blockers)
   C. Neurologic disease
      1. Cerebrovascular disease
      2. Pseudobulbar palsy
      3. Multiple sclerosis
      4. Amyotrophic lateral sclerosis
      5. Bulbar poliomyelitis
      6. Parkinsonism
   D. Muscle disease
      1. Myotonic dystrophy
      2. Muscular dystrophy
      3. Myasthenia gravis (motor end-plate)
   E. Infection
      1. Chagas' disease (Trypanosoma cruzi)
      2. Diphtheria
      3. Tetanus
   F. Metabolic
      1. Diabetes
      2. Alcoholism
      3. Thyrotoxicosis
      4. Myxedema
   G. Miscellaneous
      1. Idiopathic intestinal pseudo-obstruction
      2. Amyloidosis

Reference: Greenberger NJ. *Gastrointestinal disorders: a pathophysiological approach*, ed 4. Chicago, 1989, Year Book Medical Publishers, p. 32.

III-2 ACHALASIA

I. Pathophysiology
   A. Denervation: neuropathology of achalasia
      1. Absence or degeneration of esophageal myenteric ganglion cells
      2. Vagus nerve electron-microscopic alterations: break in continuity of axon-Schwann membranes; swelling of axons; fragmentation of neurofilaments; mitochondrial degeneration in axoplasma.
      3. Vagal nucleus: decrease in dorsal motor cells; cytologic distortion of remaining cells
   B. Functional neuropharmacology
      1. Excessive motor response of the distal esophagus to cholinergic drugs
      2. Supersensitivity of lower esophageal sphincter to gastrin (gastrin acidification) produces reduction in elevated lower esophageal tone to baseline
      3. Other factors: emotional stress, heredity

II. Clinical features
   A. Symptoms: dysphagia for liquids and solids; odynophagia occasionally; regurgitation; tracheobronchial aspiration with pulmonary changes
   B. Signs: weight loss; halitosis; occasionally signs of pulmonary inflammation

III. Diagnosis
   A. Radiography: esophageal dilatation; distal esophagus terminates in a "beak"; aperistalsis; stasis
   B. Esophageal manometry; upper sphincter normal; aperistalsis in body of esophagus; failure of lower esophageal sphincter to relax completely; elevated lower esophageal sphincter resting pressure; hypersensitivity of lower esophageal sphincter to cholinergic drugs
   C. Esophagoscopy: exclude carcinoma, benign stricture; esophageal dilatation; esophagitis

IV. Treatment
   A. Brusque dilatation: forceful dilatation of inferior sphincter with pneumatic or hydrostatic balloon dilator; satisfactory results in 60-75%
   B. Surgical therapy: distal esophageal myotomy; satisfactory results in 80%

Reference: Greenberger NJ. *Gastrointestinal disorders: a pathophysiological approach*, ed 4. Chicago, 1989, Year Book Medical Publishers, p. 33.

III-3 CONDITIONS ASSOCIATED WITH HYPERGASTRINEMIA AND DIAGNOSIS OF ZOLLINGER-ELLISON SYNDROME (ZES)

I. Conditions associated with hypergastrinemia
   A. With acid hypersecretion
      1. Gastrinoma (ZES)
      2. Antral G-cell hyperplasia
      3. Isolated retained gastric antrum
      4. Massive small intestinal resection
      5. Hyperparathyroidism
      6. Pyloric outlet obstruction
   B. With variable acid secretion
      1. Hyperthyroidism
      2. Chronic renal failure
      3. Pheochromocytoma
   C. With acid hyposecretion
      1. Pernicious anemia
      2. Atrophic gastritis
      3. Gastric carcinoma
      4. After vagotomy and pyloroplasty
II. Serum gastrin levels in ZES
   A. > 1000 pg/ml with $\uparrow$ [H$^+$] secretion - virtually diagnostic of ZES
   B. 500-1000 pg/ml — strongly suggestive of ZES
   C. 200-500 pg/ml — equivocal; 40% of patients with ZES have a gastrin level in this range
III. Provocative test for ZES
   A. Secretin injection (2 units/kg/I.V.) $\rightarrow \uparrow$ in serum gastrin > 200 pg/ml (positive in 90-95% of ZES patients)

Reference: Greenberger NJ. *Gastrointestinal disorders: a pathophysiological approach*, ed 4. Chicago, 1989, Year Book Medical Publishers, p. 98.

III-4 DIFFERENTIAL DIAGNOSIS OF REFRACTORY DUODENAL ULCERATION

I. Causes of refractory duodenal ulceration (defined as persistence of ulceration after 8 weeks treatment)
   A. Noncompliance
   B. Truly intractable duodenal ulceration
   C. Smoking
   D. *Helicobacter pylori**
   E. Continued use of aspirin and NSAIDs
   F. Gastric acid hypersecretion
      1. Zollinger-Ellison syndrome
      2. Antral G-cell hyperplasia/hyperfunction
      3. Systemic mastocytosis
   G. Stress
   H. Pyloric outlet obstruction (incomplete)
   I. Other causes of duodenal ulceration
      1. Crohn's disease
      2. Lymphoma
      3. Primary (duodenal) or secondary (pancreatic) carcinoma
      4. Tuberculosis

II. Causes of postoperative recurrent ulceration
   A. Incomplete vagotomy
   B. Zollinger-Ellison syndrome
   C. Antral G-cell hyperplasia/hyperfunction
   D. Adjacent nonabsorbable suture
   E. Retained antrum syndrome
   F. Obstruction/delayed gastric emptying
   G. Ulcerogenic drugs

*Especially important in recurrence of duodenal ulcers

III-5 DELAYED GASTRIC EMPTYING

I. Gastric retention due to pyloric outlet obstruction
   A. Chronic duodenal ulcer diseases
   B. Idiopathic hypertrophic pyloric stenosis
   C. Crohn's disease of the stomach and/or duodenum
   D. Eosinophilic gastroenteritis
   E. Carcinoma of the stomach
   F. Carcinoma of the duodenum or pancreas

II. Acute gastric retention due to mechanical obstruction
   A. Pain
      1. Renal colic
      2. Biliary colic
      3. Recent surgery
   B. Trauma
      1. Retroperitoneal hematoma
      2. Ruptured spleen
      3. Urinary tract injury
   C. Inflammation and infection
      1. Pancreatitis
      2. Peritonitis
      3. Appendicitis
      4. Sepsis
      5. Acute viral gastroenteritis
   D. Immobilization
      1. Body plaster casts
      2. Paraplegia
      3. Postoperative states
   E. Acute gastric retention due to metabolic and electrolyte abnormalities
      1. Diabetic ketoacidosis
      2. Alcoholic ketoacidosis
      3. Myxedema
      4. Acute porphyria
      5. Hepatic coma
      6. Hypokalemia
      7. Hypocalcemia
      8. Hypercalcemia

III. Chronic gastric retention
   A. Neural and smooth muscle disorders
      1. Bulbar poliomyelitis
      2. Brain tumor
      3. Demyelinating diseases (multiple sclerosis)
      4. Vagotomy usually with prior gastric surgery
      5. Scleroderma
      6. Idiopathic intestinal pseudo-obstruction

III-5 DELAYED GASTRIC EMPTYING (CONTINUED)

B. Metabolic disorders
  1. Diabetes mellitus (vagal neuropathy may be present)
  2. Myxedema
  3. Drugs
      a. Anticholinergics
      b. Opiates (morphine, codeine, etc.)
      c. Ganglionic blockers
      d. Aluminum-containing antacids
      e. Pectin and ?psyllium hydrophilic mucilloids
  4. Psychiatric disease
      a. Anorexia nervosa
  5. Idiopathic
      a. Antecedent viral illnesses

Reference: Greenberger NJ. *Gastrointestinal disorders: a pathophysiological approach*, ed 4. Chicago, 1989, Year Book Medical Publishers, p. 113.

III-6 DIAGNOSIS OF ANOREXIA NERVOSA

  I. Age of onset before 25 yr
 II. Anorexia with weight loss > 25% of original body weight
III. Distorted, implacable attitude toward eating, food, or weight that overrides hunger, admonitions, reassurance, and threats, e.g.:
  A. Denial of illness with failure to recognize nutritional needs
  B. Enjoyment in losing weight
  C. Desired body image of extreme thinness with evidence that it is rewarding to achieve and maintain this state
  D. Unusual hoarding or handling of food
 IV. No known medical illness to account for anorexia and weight loss
  V. No other psychiatric disorder
 VI. At least two of the following:
  A. Amenorrhea
  B. Lanugo
  C. Bradycardia
  D. Overactivity
  E. Bulimia
  F. Vomiting (may be self-induced)

Reference: Drossmam D, et al. *Gastroenterology* 77:1117, 1979.

III-7 CLASSIFICATION OF THE MALABSORPTION SYNDROMES

I. Inadequate digestion
   A. Postgastrectomy steatorrhea*
   B. Deficiency or inactivation of pancreatic lipase
      1. Exocrine pancreatic insufficiency
         a. Chronic pancreatitis
         b. Pancreatic carcinoma
         c. Cystic fibrosis
         d. Pancreatic resection
      2. Ulcerogenic tumor of the pancreas (Zollinger-Ellison syndrome*)
II. Reduced intestinal bile salt concentration (with impaired formation of micellar lipid)
   A. Liver disease
      1. Parenchymal liver disease
      2. Cholestasis (intrahepatic or extrahepatic)
   B. Abnormal bacterial proliferation in the small bowel
      1. Afferent loop stasis
      2. Strictures
      3. Fistulas
      4. Blind loops
      5. Multiple diverticula of the small bowel
      6. Hypomotility states (diabetes, scleroderma); intestinal pseudo-obstruction
   C. Interrupted enterohepatic circulation of bile salts
      1. Ileal resection
      2. Ileal inflammatory disease (regional ileitis)
   D. Drug-induced (by sequestration or precipitation of bile salts)
      1. Neomycin
      2. Calcium carbonate
      3. Cholestyramine
III. Inadequate absorptive surface
   A. Intestinal resection or bypass
      1. Mesenteric vascular disease with massive intestinal resection
      2. Regional enteritis with multiple bowel resection
      3. Jejunoileal bypass
   B. Gastroileostomy
IV. Lymphatic obstruction
   A. Intestinal lymphangiectasia
   B. Whipple's disease*
   C. Lymphoma*
   D. Kohlmeier-Degos (primary progressive arterial occlusive disease)*

III-7 CLASSIFICATION OF THE MALABSORPTION SYNDROME (CONTINUED)

    A. Constrictive pericarditis
    B. Congestive heart failure
    C. Mesenteric vascular insufficiency
    D. Collagen vascular disease

VI. Endocrine and metabolic disorders
    A. Diabetes mellitus
    B. Hypoparathyroidism
    C. Adrenal insufficiency
    D. Hyperthyroidism
    E. Ulcerogenic tumor of the pancreas (Zollinger-Ellison syndrome*)
    F. Carcinoid syndrome

VII. Primary mucosal absorptive defects
    A. Inflammatory or infiltrative disorders
       1. Regional enteritis*
       2. Amyloidosis
       3. Scleroderma*
       4. Lymphoma*
       5. Eosinophilic enteritis
       6. Tropical sprue
       7. Infectious enteritis (e.g., salmonellosis)
       8. Mucosal lesions associated with intestinal bacterial growth
    B. Biochemical or genetic abnormalities
       1. Celiac sprue
       2. Abetalipoproteinemia
       3. Hartnup disease
       4. Cystinuria
       5. Hypogammaglobulinemia

*Multiple mechanisms responsible for malabsorption

III-8 DIAGNOSIS OF CELIAC SPRUE

I. Evidence of malabsorption
   A. Isolated or generalized
      1. ↓ D-xylose, steatorrhea, ↓ Ca^{++}, Fe^{++}. albumin, choles-
         terol, carotenes, B_{12} absorption, ↑ protime, etc.
II. Abnormal small bowel mucosal biopsy
III. Improvement (clinical, laboratory tests, intestinal histology) with gluten-free diet
IV. Exacerbation of symptoms, diarrhea, and steatorrhea with gluten challenge
   A. Should be used only in equivocal cases

III-9 CELIAC SPRUE — FAILURE TO RESPOND TO GLUTEN-FREE DIET

I. Incorrect diagnosis
II. Nonadherence to gluten-free diet
III. Unsuspected concurrent disease such as pancreatic insufficiency
IV. Development of intestinal lymphoma
V. Development of diffuse intestinal ulceration
VI. Presence of nongranulomatous ulcerative jejunoileitis
VII. Presence of diffuse collagen deposits, i.e., "collagenous sprue"
VIII. Presence of lymphocytic (microscopic) colitis

III-10 CONDITIONS ASSOCIATED WITH BACTERIAL OVERGROWTH

I. Billroth II subtotal gastrectomy with afferent loop stasis
II. Blind loops
III. Multiple small bowel diverticula
IV. Hypomotility states (diabetes, scleroderma, intestinal pseudo-obstruction)
V. Incomplete small bowel obstruction
VI. Gastric achlorhydria (pernicious anemia)
VII. Strictures (regional enteritis, radiation injury)
VIII. Fistulas (regional enteritis)

III-11 DIAGNOSIS OF "BACTERIAL OVERGROWTH" SYNDROME

*I. Steatorrhea — usually moderate (15-30 gm/day)
II. D-xylose — can be normal or abnormal
III. Small bowel biopsy — can be normal or abnormal
*IV. Vitamin B_{12} absorption with I.F.
*V. (+) Small bowel culture
   A. Usually > 10^7 organisms/ml
   B. Polymicrobial (E. coli, bacteroides, enterococci, anaerobic lactobacilli)
VI. Abnormal breath tests (lactulose, ^{14}C-xylose, etc.)

* Correction of #1, 4, and 5 with antibiotic therapy

III-12 CLINICAL FEATURES OF ZINC DEFICIENCY

Skin
- Acrodermatitis enteropathica
- Alopecia
- Poor wound healing

Neuropsychiatric
- Depression
- Irritability
- Lack of concentration
- Tremor

Eyes
- Night blindness

Gastrointestinal
- Anorexia
- Impaired taste
- Diarrhea

Pancreatic insufficiency

Endocrine
- Hypogonadism
- Dwarfism in children
- Insulin hypersensitivity

Reference: Tasman-Jones C. In Stollerman G, editor: *Advances in internal medicine*, vol 26. Chicago, 1980, Year Book Medical Publishers, p. 105.

III-13 DIFFERENTIAL DIAGNOSIS OF REGIONAL ENTERITIS

I. Infectious enteritis (bacterial, fungal, protozoal)
   A. Must exclude amebiasis, campylobacter, yersinia, chlamydia
II. Tuberculous enteritis
III. Lymphoma
IV. Carcinoid tumor
V. Carcinoma
VI. Intestinal lymphangiectasia
VII. Ischemic small bowel disease with/without segmental infarcts
   A. Connective tissue disease with vasculitis (PN, SLE)
   B. Atherosclerotic/embolic disease
VIII. Malabsorptive disorders with primary gut involvement
   A. Celiac sprue
   B. Amyloidosis
   C. Whipple's disease
IX. Nongranulomatous ulcerative jejunoileitis
X. Eosinophilic gastroenteritis
XI. Nonsteroidal antiinflammatory drugs (NSAIDs)

III-14 FEATURES DIFFERENTIATING IDIOPATHIC ULCERATIVE COLITIS FROM GRANULOMATOUS COLITIS*

Features	Ulcerative colitis	Granulomatous colitis
I. CLINICAL FEATURES		
Diarrhea	+ + + +	+ + +
Hematochezia	+ + + +	+ +
Abdominal tenderness	+ +	+ + +
Abdominal mass	0	+ + to + + +
Toxic megacolon	+	+
Perforation	+	+
Fistulas		
Perianal, perineal	0	+ +
Enteroenteric	0	+
II. ENDOSCOPIC FEATURES (sigmoidoscopy, colonoscopy)		
Rectal involvement	+ + + +	+ +
Diffuse, continuous disease	+ + + +	+
Friability, purulence	+ + + to + + +	+
Aphthous, linear ulcers	0	+ + + to + + + +
Cobblestoning	0	+ + to + + +
Pseudopolyps	+ +	+
III. RADIOLOGIC FEATURES		
Continuous disease	+ + + +	0 to +
Associated ileal disease	0	+ +
Strictures	0	+ to + +
Fistulas	0	+ to + +
Asymmetric wall involvement	0	+ + to + + +
Fissures	0	+ to + +
IV. PATHOLOGIC FEATURES		
Granulomas	0	+ + + to + + + +
Transmural inflammation	0 to +	+ + + to + + + +
Crypt abscess	+ + +	+ to + +
Skip areas of involvement	+	+ + +
Linear, aphthous ulcers	0	+ + + to + + + +

*Key: 0 = never or rarely; + = < 25%; + + = 25-50%; + + + = 50-75%; + + + + = > 75%

Reference: Greenberger NJ. *Gastrointestinal disorders: a pathophysiological approach*, ed 4. Chicago, 1989, Year Book Medical Publishers, p. 226.

III-15 SYSTEMIC MANIFESTATIONS OF ULCERATIVE COLITIS (UC) AND REGIONAL ENTERITIS (RE)

	UC	RE
I. Skin		
A. Erythema nodosum	+	+
B. Pyoderma gangrenosum	+	+
C. Ulcerating erythematous plaques	+	+
II. Eyes		
A. Uveitis	+	+
III. Mouth		
A. Aphthous ulcers, cheilitis	±	+
IV. Esophagus		
A. Ulceration	+	+
V. Stomach and duodenum		
A. Pyloric outlet obstruction	—	+
VI. Small bowel		
A. Malabsorption	—	+
B. Lactose intolerance	+	+
VII. Liver		
A. Steatosis	+	+
B. Cirrhosis	+	+
C. Chronic active liver disease	+	+
D. Granulomas	—	+
VIII. Gallbladder and biliary tree		
A. Cholelithiasis	—	+
B. Sclerosing cholangitis	+	rarely present
C. Bile duct carcinoma	+	—
IX. Renal disease		
A. Obstructive hydronephrosis	—	+
B. Nephrolithiasis	+(urate)	+(oxalate)
X. Anemia		
A. Blood loss	+	+
B. Hemolysis	+	+
C. Folate depletion (sulfasalazine)	+	+
D. Chronic illness	+	+
XI. Thrombocytosis	+	+
XII. Pulmonary		
A. Fibrosing alveolitis	+	—
B. Pulmonary vasculitis	+	—
XIII. Pancreatitis		
A. Ductal obstruction	—	+
B. Drugs (azathioprine, sulfasalazine, steroids)	+	+
XIV. Vulva (Crohn's disease)	—	+
XV. Joints		
A. Arthritis	+	+

III-16 DIAGNOSIS OF IRRITABLE BOWEL SYNDROME

I. Criteria useful in establishing the diagnosis
  A. Usual criteria
    1. Symptoms: abdominal pain, diarrhea, alternating diarrhea and constipation, relief of abdominal pain with defecation, feeling of incomplete evacuation with defecation, absence of nocturnal symptoms
    2. Absence of systemic symptoms: anorexia, weight loss, fever, and signs, i.e., anemia
    3. No hematochezia, melena, or occult blood in stool
    4. Normal sigmoidoscopy
    5. Normal barium enema
  B. Additional criteria if symptoms persist
    1. Normal stool weight (24 hr stool weight < 300 gm)
    2. No steatorrhea or evidence of malabsorption
    3. Normal upper gastrointestinal tract and small bowel x-ray films
II. Differential diagnosis
  A. Lactose intolerance
  B. Other disaccharidase deficiencies, i.e., sucrose-isomaltose intolerance
  C. Subclinical carbohydrate malabsorption
  D. Diverticular and "prediverticular disease"
  E. Drug-induced diarrhea
  F. Idiopathic bile acid malabsorption
  G. Inadvertent dietary indiscretion (excess caffeine, tea, cola beverages, etc.)
  H. Irritable bowel disorder not associated with an underlying disorder
  I. Motility disorders small bowel or colon (incompletely defined)

III-17 CLASSIFICATION, DIAGNOSIS AND MANAGEMENT OF CHRONIC DIARRHEAL DISORDERS

Cause	Examples	Key elements in diagnosis	Treatment
1. Iatrogenic dietary factors	Excess tea, coffee, cola beverages, simple sugars	Careful history taking	Appropriate dietary modifications
2. Infectious enteritis	Amebiasis Giardiasis	Demonstrate leukocytes in stool Identify trophozoites or cysts in stool and duodenal aspirate (giardiasis)	Amebiasis—metronidazole diodoquin antibiotics Giardiasis—metronidazole
3. Inflammatory bowel disease	Ulcerative colitis Regional enteritis	History: Diarrhea, abdominal pain, rectal bleeding Sigmoidoscopy, barium enema, UGI, and small bowel series	Sulfasalazine Corticosteroids
4. Irritable bowel syndrome	See Table III-16	See Table III-16 Antispasmodics	Dietary modifications
5. Incontinence	Diabetes Rectal surgery Radiation proctitis	History	Depends on cause
6. Idiopathic secretory		Stool output > 1.0 L/24 hr, No ↓ stool volume with fasting, Stool osmolality gap ≤ 40 mOsm/kg	

III-17 CLASSIFICATION, DIAGNOSIS AND MANAGEMENT OF CHRONIC DIARRHEAL DISORDERS (CONTINUED)

Cause	Examples	Key elements in diagnosis	Treatment
7. Lactose intolerance	Milk intolerance	Milk → abdominal pain, diarrhea, gas, bloating. Cessation of milk drinking → amelioration of symptoms. Lactose load (1 gm/kg) → exacerbation of symptoms and breath H_2 fails to rise	Discontinue milk
8. Laxative abuse		Add few drops of NaOH to stool. Because most laxatives contain phenolphthalein, the stool will turn red.	Discontinue laxative
9. Drug-induced	Antacids, antibiotics (clindamycin, ampicillin, penicillin), NSAIDs, colchicine, lactulose, sorbitol	Careful history taking and review of medication.	Discontinue offending drug
10. Diverticular and pre-diverticular disease		History: intermittent symptoms PE: Palpable LF. colon Barium enema: diverticulosis and/or muscle hypertrophy	High fiber diet. Avoid: corn, nuts, peanuts, kernel-containing foods.

III-17 CLASSIFICATION, DIAGNOSIS AND MANAGEMENT OF CHRONIC DIARRHEAL DISORDERS (CONTINUED)

Cause	Examples	Key elements in diagnosis	Treatment
11. Malabsorptive disease	Pancreatic insufficiency Regional enteritis Short bowel Bacterial overgrowth	UGI plus small bowel x-rays; tests of intestinal absorptive function: D-xylose, stool fat, Schilling test, serum carotenes, calcium, albumin, cholesterol, iron, prothrombin time	Appropriate for the underlying disorder
12. Metabolic	Diabetes mellitus Hyperthyroidism Adrenal insufficiency	Abnormal blood glucose levels ↑T$_4$, ↓TSH, ↑RAI uptake ↓plasma cortisol, ↓response to synthetic ACTH	Appropriate for the underlying disorder
13. Mechanical	Fecal impaction	Rectal examination	Remove impaction
14. Neoplastic	Carcinoma of the pancreas Carcinoid syndrome Villous adenoma Medullary carcinoma of the thyroid Tumors producing V.I.P. (vasoactive intestinal peptide) Gastrinoma	Suspect the diagnosis	Surgical
15. Postoperative history	Gastric surgery Intestinal resection (especially ileum) Short bowel syndrome		

III-18 RISK FACTORS FOR DEVELOPING COLON CANCER

    I. Age > 40 years
   II. Family history of colon cancer
  III. Prior colon carcinoma
  IV. Familial polyposis
   V. Gardner's syndrome
  VI. Villous adenoma
 VII. Colonic polyps (especially if > 2 cm)
VIII. Idiopathic ulcerative colitis
  IX. Granulomatous colitis (Crohn's disease)
   X. Prior breast or female genital tract cancer
  XI. Asbestosis
 XII. Diet rich in beef and lipid (controversial)
XIII. Acromegaly (data incomplete)
XIV. Peutz-Jeghers syndrome
 XV. Postcholecystectomy (controversial)

Reference: Greenberger NJ. *Gastrointestinal disorders: a pathophysiological approach*, ed 4. Chicago, 1989, Year Book Medical Publishers, p. 240.

III-19 DIAGNOSIS OF CHRONIC ALCOHOLISM

I. Evidence of alcohol withdrawal syndromes
   A. Tremulousness
   B. Alcoholic hallucinosis
   C. Withdrawal seizures or "rum fits"
   D. Delirium tremens
II. Evidence of tolerance to alcohol
   A. Ingestion of 1 fifth or more of whiskey per day
   B. No gross evidence of intoxication with blood alcohol level > 150 mg/100 ml
   C. Random blood alcohol level > 300 mg/100 ml
   D. Accelerated clearance of blood alcohol (> 25 mg/100 ml per hour)
III. Psychosociologic factors
   A. Continued ingestion of alcohol despite strong contraindication to do so:
      1. Threatened loss of job
      2. Threatened loss of spouse and/or family
      3. Medical contraindication known to patient
   B. Admission of inability to discontinue use of alcohol
IV. Presence of alcohol-associated disorders
   A. Erosive gastritis with upper gastrointestinal bleeding
   B. Pancreatitis, acute and chronic, in the absence of cholelithiasis
   C. Alcoholic liver disease (fatty liver, alcoholic hepatitis, cirrhosis)
   D. Alcoholic diseases of the nervous system
      1. Peripheral neuropathy
      2. Cerebellar degeneration
      3. Wernicke-Korsakoff syndrome
      4. Beriberi
      5. Alcoholic myopathy
      6. Alcoholic cardiomyopathy
V. "CAGE" criteria
   A. C = Concerned about drinking
   B. A = Annoyed about questions on drinking
   C. G = Guilty about drinking
   D. E = Eye opener, i.e., morning drink needed

Reference: Kaim SC, et al. Ann Int Med 77:249, 1972.

III-20 SPECTRUM OF ALCOHOLIC LIVER DISEASE

I. Alcoholic fatty liver
   A. Clear cytoplasmic vacuoles
   B. Eccentrically placed cell nuclei
II. Alcoholic hepatitis
   A. Polymorphonuclear infiltration
   B. Alcoholic hyaline
   C. Central hyaline necrosis and sclerosis of central vein
   D. Fat and/or fibrosis may be present
III. Alcoholic cirrhosis
   A. Distortion of lobular architecture
   B. Fibrous septa involving portal and central zones
IV. Secondary changes
   A. Cholestasis
   B. Bile duct proliferation
   C. Siderosis
   D. Fat

III-21 CLINICAL AND HISTOLOGICAL FEATURES OF ALCOHOLIC HEPATITIS

I. Clinical features
   A. General considerations: Spectrum of clinical findings ranging from asymptomatic to florid decompensated liver disease with hepatosplenomegaly, jaundice, ascites, azotemia, and encephalopathy
   B. Symptoms: Anorexia, weakness, abdominal pain, weight loss, fever
   C. Signs: Jaundice, peripheral stigmata of chronic liver disease, hepatomegaly, splenomegaly, ascites, edema, signs of hepatic encephalopathy
   D. Laboratory data: ↑MCV, ↑WBC, ↑SGOT, ↑SGOT:SGPT (AST:ALT) > 3:1, ↑bilirubin, ↓albumin, prolonged prothrombin time
   E. Histologic features of alcoholic hepatitis
      1. Absolute criteria
         a. Hepatocellular necrosis
         b. Polymorphonuclear infiltration of the liver
      2. Generally accepted criteria
         a. Mallory alcoholic hyaline
      3. Often present but not required for the diagnosis
         a. Fatty infiltration of the liver
         b. Fibrosis
         c. Cirrhosis

III-21 CLINICAL AND HISTOLOGICAL FEATURES OF ALCOHOLIC HEPATITIS (CONTINUED)

    F. Diagnosis of alcoholic hepatitis
1. History of excessive alcohol intake
2. Liver biopsy showing changes of alcoholic hepatitis
3. Lab: ↑MCV, ↑SGOT, ↑GGTP, ↑SGOT:SGPT ratio

    G. Indicators of a bad prognosis
1. Serum bilirubin > 20 mg/dl
2. BUN > 25 mg/dl without obvious cause
3. Hepatic encephalopathy
4. Prothrombin time prolonged > 6 seconds compared to controls

III-22 HEPATITIS A

  I. General considerations
    A. Short incubation period (14-24 days)
    B. Fecal-oral transmission (epidemics with contaminated water)
    C. Virus present in stools from incubation period to onset of clinical illness
    D. Triad of headache, fever, myalgias favors hepatitis A over hepatitis B
    E. Maximum period of infectivity 2 weeks after onset of clinical illness
    F. Frequently anicteric
    G. Does not result in chronic liver disease
    H. Infection confers immunity

  II. Immunologic considerations
    A. Hepatitis A antigen (HA Ag) circulates transiently at low titers
    B. HA Ag cleared rapidly from stool
    C. HA Ag detection in serum and stool not feasible clinically
    D. HA Ab rises rapidly, peaks after 2-3 months, persists
  *E. HA Ab in acute phase is IgM; later ($\geq$4 months) is IgG
    F. HA Ab present in majority of adults (> 50% at age > 60)
    G. Conventional immune serum globulin *modifies* the disease

*IgM antibody persists for > 120 days in > 10% of patients

Reference: Greenberger NJ. *Gastrointestinal disorders: a pathophysiological approach*, ed 4. Chicago, 1989, Year Book Medical Publishers, p. 317.

III-23 HEPATITIS C

I. General information
   A. 1-2 million cases in the U.S., majority not diagnosed
   B. Estimated 100,000 new cases/year with 2nd generation screening tests
   C. Incubation period 6-14 weeks (mean, 7-8)
   D. Hepatitis C antigen demonstrable in liver
   E. Virus characteristics by electron microscopy similar to hepatitis B virus

II. Role of hepatitis C in liver disease
   A. Acute hepatitis
   B. Chronic hepatitis (50% to 60% of population with acute hepatitis C)
   C. Cirrhosis (20% to 25% of patients with acute hepatitis C)
   D. Alcoholic liver disease (hepatitis C may potentiate development)
   E. Hepatocellular carcinoma (25% to 60% test HCV positive)

III. Epidemiologic settings
   A. Transfusion associated (acute as well as remote)
   B. Parenteral drug abuse
   C. Transplant patients
   D. Multiply transfused hemophiliacs
   E. Hemodialysis patients
   F. Prisoners; institutionalized individuals
   G. Health care workers
   H. Tattoos, shared razors, shared toothbrushes
   I. High risk sexual behavior (multiple partners)
   J. Unknown risk factors identified (40% to 50% cases)

IV. Clinical factors
   A. Patient often asymptomatic and frequently detected by elevated serum aminotransferase
   B. Histologic changes of chronic hepatitis/cirrhosis may not correlate with physical findings or liver test abnormalities
   C. 2nd generation test for hepatitis C virus (HCV-antibody) positive in 85% to 90% patients with acute hepatitis C.
   D. Evidence of hepatitis C infection (either HCV antibody or HCV-RNA) persists for many years after infection
   E. Disease can be latent for many years

V. Treatment
   A. Interferon alpha 2B given for 6 months results in clinical response in 50% of patients, half of whom relapse within 6 months.

III-24 HEPATITIS B

Epidemiologic considerations

Long incubation period (50-180 days)
Transmitted by parenteral and nonparenteral routes
HB_sAg: spheres, tubules, Dane particles
Spheres and tubules represent viral surface coat material made in infected hepatocytes
Dane particle contains inner core antigen (HB_cAg) and outer shell (HB_sAg) and represents complete virion
HB_sAg detected in blood, saliva, urine, semen, breast milk, bile
Sexual partners, homosexuals, and newborn infants have high rate of infection

Immunologic considerations

Antigen	Significance	Antibody	Significance
HB_sAg	Hepatitis B infection	Anti-HB_s (HB_sAb)	Denotes prior hepatitis B infection and usually immunity
HB_cAg	Hepatitis B infection	Anti-HB_c (HB_cAb)	Recent or ongoing infection HB_sAg carriers — high titers
DNA polymerase HB_cAg	High infectivity; viral replication Suggests high infectivity; associated with active disease	Anti-HB_c (HB_cAb)	Suggests limited/no disease activity and low-grade infectivity
Delta antigen	Infection with Delta agent	Delta antibody	Accelerated course of chronic hepatitis; increased risk of fulminant hepatitis

III-24 HEPATITIS B (CONTINUED)

Diagnosis of Hepatitis B (HBV) Infection

HB_sAg positive in 75-85% of HBV infections
Reasons:
HBV present but below detectable concentrations
HBV cleared, no HB_sAb (serologic window)
DX in HB_sAg negative patients established by demonstrating HB_sAb
(+) HB_sAg or other HBV markers in 30-40% chronic active liver disease patients

Spectrum of responses in hepatitis B infections

Acute icteric hepatitis
Serum bilirubin > 3.0 mg/dl
Serum transaminases > 100 on > 2 occasions 4 days apart
Acute anicteric hepatitis
Serum bilirubin < 3.0 mg/dl
Serum transaminases > 100 on > 2 occasions 4 days apart
Seroconversion with HB_sAg positivity
$HB_sAg \rightarrow HB_sAb$
Seroconversion without HB_sAg positivity
HB_sAb (-) $\rightarrow HB_sAb$ (+)

III-24 HEPATITIS B (CONTINUED)

Interpretation of serological abnormalities in hepatitis B infection

	Tests			Interpretations
	HB_sAg	HB_cAb	HB_sAb	
1.	+	−	−	a. Acute viral hepatitis
2.	+	+	−	a. Acute viral hepatitis b. Chronic active hepatitis or Chronic persistent hepatitis c. Chronic carrier state
3.	−	+	−	a. Acute viral hepatitis (in window phase) b. Remote B viral infection
4.	−	+	+	a. Remote B viral infection b. Chronic hepatitis in immunosuppressed patient (HB_sAb titer is usually low) c. Subclinical infection
5.	−	−	+	a. Remote B viral infection b. Immunization response
6.	+	−	+	a. Remote and recent B viral infection

Reference: Greenberger NJ. *Gastrointestinal disorders: a pathophysiological approach*, ed 4. Chicago, 1989, Year Book Medical Publishers, pp. 318-319.

III-25 ETIOLOGY AND DIAGNOSIS OF CHRONIC ACTIVE LIVER DISEASE

I. Causes of chronic active liver disease
   A. Autoimmune
   B. Viral hepatitis, type B
   C. Viral hepatitis, non-A, non-B (hepatitis C)
   D. Drugs
      *1. Alpha-methyldopa
      2. Aspirin (esp. in patients with rheumatoid arthritis)
      3. Acetaminophen
      4. Allopurinol
      5. Halothane
      *6. Isoniazid
      *7. Nitrofurantoin
      8. Oxyphenisatin
      9. Propylthiouracil
      10. Sulfonamides
      11. Interferon Alpha 2B
   E. Miscellaneous
      1. Wilson's disease
      2. Alpha-1-antitrypsin disease
      3. Alcohol
II. Diagnosis of chronic active liver disease†
   A. Persistence of symptoms and signs of liver disease for > 6 months
   B. Persistence of abnormal liver tests for > 6 months
      1. ↑ Aminotransferase
      2. ↑ Gammaglobulins
   C. Abnormal hepatic histology
      1. Chronic active hepatitis without cirrhosis
         a. Periportal and piecemeal necrosis with portal zone expansion and rosette formation
         b. Multilobular necrosis
         c. Bridging (confluent) hepatic necrosis
         d. Periportal plus piecemeal necrosis
      2. Chronic active hepatitis with cirrhosis

*most important
†Demonstration of ongoing activity for at least 6 *months* emphasizes the unresolving nature of the process and is desirable for establishing the diagnosis. However, the onset of illness may be difficult to estimate. Thus, patients with disease of less than 6 months duration may develop hypoalbuminemia, hypergammaglobulinemia, and ascites and yet the disease is not fully chronic as judged by international criteria.

References: Boyer JL. *Gastroenterology* 70:1161, 1976, and Czaja AJ. *Mayo Clin Proc* 56:311, 1981.

III-26 PRIMARY BILIARY CIRRHOSIS

I. Diagnosis
   A. Hepatomegaly
   B. ↑ Serum alkaline phosphatase
   C. (+) test for antimitochondrial antibody
   D. ↑ IgM levels
   E. ↑ Serum cholesterol
   F. Compatible histologic changes on liver biopsy
   G. Exclusion of extrahepatic obstruction

II. Natural history of primary biliary cirrhosis
   A. Hepatomegaly
   B. Pruritus
   C. Increased pigmentation
   D. Hyperbilirubinemia
   E. Xanthomata
   F. Splenomegaly
   G. Ascites
   H. GI bleeding
   I. Encephalopathy

Appearance of clinical features as course of the disease progresses

III. Liver transplantation

III-27 COMMON PRECIPITATING CAUSES OF HEPATIC ENCEPHALOPATHY

Causes	Possible mechanisms leading to coma
I. Azotemia (spontaneous or induced diuresis)	↑BUN leads to ↑endogenous NH_3 production; direct suppressive effect on brain from uremia
II. Sedatives, tranquilizers, anesthetics	Direct depressive effect on brain; impaired metabolism of sedative drugs with hepatic parenchymal cell failure
III. Gastrointestinal hemorrhage	Provides substrate for increased NH_3 production (100 ml blood = 15-20 gm protein) Shock and hypoxia Hypovolemia → impaired cerebral, hepatic, and renal function Azotemia can lead to further ↑ in blood NH_3 due to load of NH_3 from transfused blood (Storage at 4°C: 1 day = 170 mg/100 ml; 4 days = 330; 21 days = 900.)
IV. Diuretics	Induce ↓K^+ alkalosis ↓K^+ leads to ↑renal output NH_3 across blood-brain barrier Vigorous diuresis can result in hypovolemia and impaired cardiac, cerebral, hepatic, and renal function, the latter resulting in azotemia; azotemia ↑endogenous NH_3 production
V. Metabolic alkalosis	Favors transfer of nonionized NH_3 across blood-brain barrier
VI. Increased dietary protein intake	Provides substrate for increased NH_3 production

III-27 COMMON PRECIPITATING CAUSES OF HEPATIC ENCEPHALOPATHY (CONTINUED)

Causes	Possible mechanisms leading to coma
VII. Infection	↑Tissue catabolism leading to ↑endogenous NH_3 load Dehydration and impaired renal function Hypoxia, hypotension, hyperthermia may potentiate NH_3 toxicity
VIII. Constipation	Intestinal production and absorption of NH_3 and other nitrogenous products
IX. Hepatic injury	Superimposed viral or toxic parenchymal cell injury may compromise liver function
X. Miscellaneous	NH_4- containing drugs (NH_4Cl) Acquired form of renal tubular acidosis (distal type) with inappropriate kaliuresis Genetic disorders with specific deficiency of urea cycle enzymes Presence of hypoglycemia, hypercarbia, or severe hypoxemia in patients with marginal hepatocellular function

References: Schenker S. *Gastroenterology* 66:121, 1974, and Jr., et al. Hoyumpa AM. *Gastroenterology* 76:184, 1979.

III-28 DIFFERENTIAL DIAGNOSIS OF ASCITES

I. Transudative effusions
    A. Cirrhosis of the liver*
    B. Congestive heart failure*
    C. Constrictive pericarditis*
    D. Obstruction to the hepatic veins (Budd-Chiari syndrome)*
        1. Associated with tumors (hepatoma, hypernephroma, cancer of pancreas)

III-28 DIFFERENTIAL DIAGNOSIS OF ASCITES (CONTINUED)

      2. Associated with hematologic disorders) myeloproliferative disease, polycythemia vera, myeloid metaplasia)

      3. Due to infections (pylephlebitis)

  E. Obstruction to the inferior vena cava

  F. Nephrotic syndrome

  G. Viral hepatitis with submassive or massive hepatic necrosis

  H. Meig's syndrome

  I. Myelofibrosis

  J. Spontaneous bacterial peritonitis (SBP)

II. Exudative effusions

  A. Neoplastic diseases involving the peritoneum*

      1. Peritoneal carcinomatosis

      2. Lymphomatous disorders

  B. Tuberculous peritonitis*

  C. Pancreatitis* (also leaking pseudocyst and disrupted main pancreatic duct)

  D. Talc or starch powder peritonitis following surgery

  E. Transected lymphatics following portal-caval shunt surgery

  F. Myxedema

  G. Sarcoidosis

  H. Lymphatic obstruction

      1. Intestinal lymphangiectasia

      2. Lymphomas

  I. Pseudomyxoma peritonei

  J. Struma ovarii

  K. Amyloidosis

  L. Prior abdominal trauma with ruptured lymphatics

  M. Nephrogenic ascites†

  N. Primary bacterial peritonitis (PBP)

III. Disorders simulating ascites

  A. Pancreatic pseudocyst

  B. Hydronephrosis

  C. Ovarian cyst

  D. Mesenteric cyst

  E. Obesity

*Most common disorders.

†Occurs in patients with renal failure on maintenance hemodialysis.

Reference: Greenberger NJ. *Gastrointestinal disorders: a pathophysiological approach*, ed 4. Chicago, 1989, Year Book Medical Publishers, p. 367.

III-29 CONDITIONS CAUSING OR CONTRIBUTING TO POSTOPERATIVE JAUNDICE

I. Increased load of bilirubin pigment
   A. Hemolytic anemia
   B. Resorption of hematomas or hemoperitoneum
   C. Pulmonary infarction
   D. Transfusions: If blood stored > 1 week approximately 10% of red blood cells hemolyzed → extra load of ~ 7.5 gm hemoglobin. 7.5 x 35 = ~ 250 mg extra bilirubin/unit blood
II. Impaired hepatocellular function
   A. Hepatitis-like picture
      1. Posttransfusion hepatitis
         a. Hepatitis B, hepatitis C (now rare)
         b. Non-A, non-B hepatitis, non-C hepatitis
         c. Cytomegalovirus, EB virus, adenovirus, ECHO, coxsackie
      2. Hypotension
      3. Halothane anesthesia
      4. Drugs
   B. Intrahepatic cholestasis
      1. Hypotension
      2. Hypoxemia
      3. Sepsis
      4. Drugs
      5. Total parenteral nutrition
   C. Congestive heart failure
III. Extrahepatic biliary tract obstruction
   A. Bile duct injury
   B. Choledocholithiasis

Reference: LaMont JF, Isselbacher KJ. *N Engl J Med* 288:305, 1973.

III-30 DIFFERENTIAL DIAGNOSIS OF JAUNDICE DUE TO INTRAHEPATIC CHOLESTASIS*

I. Hepatocellular
   A. Viral hepatitis
   B. Alcoholic hepatitis
   C. Chronic active hepatitis
   D. Alpha-1 antitrypsin deficiency
II. Hepatocanalicular
   A. Drugs (17-alkylated steroids, phenothiazines)
   B. Sepsis
   C. Toxic shock syndrome
   D. Postoperative
   E. Total parenteral nutrition
   F. Neoplasms (Hodgkin's disease, lymphoma, prostatic carcinoma)
   G. Sickle cell anemia
   H. Amyloidosis
III. Ductular
   A. Sarcoidosis
   B. Primary biliary cirrhosis
IV. Ducts
   A. Intrahepatic biliary atresia
   B. Intrahepatic sclerosing cholangitis
   C. Caroli's disease
   D. Cholangiocarcinoma
V. Recurrent cholestasis
   A. Benign recurrent intrahepatic cholestasis
   B. Recurrent jaundice of pregnancy
   C. Dubin-Johnson syndrome

*Classification based on apparent site of hepatic injury.

III-31 DIFFERENTIAL DIAGNOSIS OF IRON STORAGE DISEASE AND CLINICAL FEATURES OF IDIOPATHIC HEMOCHROMATOSIS

	Iron overload in family members	Anemia	Cirrhosis	Transferrin saturation	Serum ferritin	Desferrioxamine iron excretion
I. Refractory anemias	0	+	0	Normal to ↑	Variable	Variable
II. Laennec's cirrhosis	0	±	+	Normal	Normal to ↑	2-4 mg/24 hr
III. Excess oral iron intake	0	±	0	↑	Normal to ↑	Variable
IV. Transfusion	0	+	0	↑	↑	Variable
V. Idiopathic hemochromatosis*	+	0	±	> 80%	> 1000 ng/ml	>8 mg/24hr

A. Skin pigmentation
B. Diabetes mellitus
C. Hepatomegaly, splenomegaly, cirrhosis
D. Hypogonadism
E. Cardiomyopathy and congestive heart failure
F. Adrenal insufficiency
G. Arthropathy

+ = present; 0 = absent; ± = may or may not be present.
* Liver biopsy shows parenchymal distribution of iron deposits.

Reference: Greenberger NJ. *Gastrointestinal disorders: a pathophysiological approach*, ed 4. Chicago, 1989, Year Book Medical Publishers, p. 388.

III-32 COMPARISON OF THE CLINICAL, RADIOLOGIC, AND PATHOLOGIC CHARACTERISTICS OF FOCAL NODULAR HYPERPLASIA AND LIVER CELL ADENOMA*

	Focal nodular hyperplasia	Liver cell adenoma
I. Clinical		
Incidence	Uncommon	Rare
Age	All ages	Third, fourth decades
Sex	85% F	Nearly all F
Oral contraceptive use	Occasionally	Nearly always
Clinical presentation	Usually asymptomatic 35% have abdominal mass, abdominal discomfort	Often abdominal emergency, 45% abdominal mass, acute abdominal pain
Hemoperitoneum	Less than 1%	25%
Liver function tests	Nearly always normal	Nearly always normal
Malignant potential	Resection if operative risk negligible	Resection
II. Angiography		
Vascularity	Hypervascular with dense capillary blush	Hypovascular
Hematoma formation	Rare	Common
Necrosis	Rare	Common
Septation	Present in 50%	Absent
III. Liver scan		
Uptake	Normal or slightly decreased	None

III-32 COMPARISON OF THE CLINICAL, RADIOLOGIC, AND PATHOLOGIC CHARACTERISTICS OF FOCAL NODULAR HYPERPLASIA AND LIVER CELL ADENOMA* (CONTINUED)

	Focal nodular hyperplasia	Liver cell adenoma
IV. Pathology		
Capsule	No capsule	Partial to ample encapsulation
Location	Usually subscapular, 20% pedunculated	Usually subscapular, 7% pedunculated
Lesions	Often multiple	Usually solitary
Stellate scar	Present	Absent
Parenchyma	Nodular	Homogenous
Hemorrhage, necrosis	Rare	Common
Bile stasis	Absent	Present
Hepatocytes	Cytologically normal	Glycogen rich, vacuolated
Bile ductules	Present	Absent
Kupffer cells	Present	Reduced or absent
Vascularity	Large thick-walled vessels	Thin-walled sinusoids
Ultrastructure	Normal	Simplified

*Modified from: Knowles DM. II, et al. *Medicine* 57:223, 1978.

III-33 CLINICAL FEATURES OF HEPATOMA

I. General
80% to 90% of primary hepatic neoplasms are hepatic cell carcinomas (i.e., hepatoma); 10% are bile duct carcinomas (cholangiocarcinoma); approximately 70% of patients have underlying cirrhosis, most frequently postnecrotic or "mixed" type

II. Symptoms
A. Common: weight loss, abdominal pain, anorexia, nausea, and emesis, which occur in 40% to 70% of patients
B. Uncommon: fever, cough, hemoptysis

III. Physical Findings
A. Common: hepatomegaly, ascites, jaundice, hepatic bruit, liver tenderness to palpation, edema

III-33 CLINICAL FEATURES OF HEPATOMA (CONTINUED)

  B. Uncommon: splenomegaly, hepatic coma (except terminally), fever
IV. Atypical Presentations and Manifestations
  A. Acute cholecystitis syndrome
  B. Acute abdominal catastrophe (hemoperitoneum)
  C. Pulmonary embolism with or without infarction and malignant pleural effusion
  D. Budd-Chiari syndrome
  E. Erythrocytosis (~10% of patients)
  F. Hypercalcemia
  G. Hyperglycemia
  H. Hypercholesterolemia
  I. Fever of unknown origin
V. Diagnosis
  A. Clinical findings
    1. Unexplained deterioration in a cirrhotic*
    2. Hepatomegaly with a disproportionately ↑ serum alkaline phosphatase with no or little elevation in serum bilirubin*
    3. Hepatic bruit
    4. Elevated right hemidiaphragm
VI. Laboratory findings
  A. Abnormal liver scan/sonogram/CT scan
  B. Abnormal hepatic angiogram*
  C. Abnormal fibrinogen
  D. Positive liver biopsy (approximately 70% of cases)*
  E. Distant metastases
VII. Serologic tumor markers
  A. Alpha-fetoprotein (70% to 85% of cases)
  B. Hepatitis B markers in serum and liver (42% to 88% of cases)
  C. Vitamin B_{12} binding protein (7% of cases)
  D. Alpha$_1$-antitrypsin (5% of cases)
  E. Hepatitis C markers (40% to 70% of cases)
VIII. Course
  A. Average course is 4-8 months after onset of symptoms
  B. Generally poor responses to chemotherapy
  C. Gastrointestinal bleeding is common (35% to 50% of cases)
  D. Hepatic coma develops in 20% to 30% of cases

*Most important

Reference: Greenberger NJ. *Gastrointestinal disorders: a pathophysiological approach*, ed 4. Chicago, 1989, Year Book Medical Publishers, p. 391.

III-34 DIAGNOSIS OF WILSON'S DISEASE

I. Abnormalities uniformly present
* A. Kayser-Fleischer rings
* B. Serum ceruloplasmin (< 20 mg/100 ml)
* C. Urine copper excretion (> 100 μg/day)
  D. Liver copper content (> 250 μg/gm dry wt. of liver)
  E. Abnormal metabolism of ^{64}Cu

II. Abnormalities frequently present
  A. ↓ Serum uric acid and uricosuria
  B. Aminoaciduria
  C. Renal glycosuria
  D. Chronic active liver disease, cirrhosis
  E. Splenomegaly
  F. Thrombocytopenia
  G. Hemolytic anemia

III. Central nervous system abnormalities

*These three items are used to screen for Wilson's disease.

Reference: Greenberger NJ. Gastrointestinal disorders: a pathophysiological approach, ed 4. Chicago, 1989, Year Book Medical Publishers, p. 390.

III-35 PRINCIPAL ALTERATIONS OF HEPATIC MORPHOLOGY PRODUCED BY SOME COMMONLY USED DRUGS AND CHEMICALS

Principal morphologic change	Class of agent	Example
Cholestasis	Anabolic steroid	Methyl testosterone*
	Antithyroid	Methimazole
	Chemotherapeutic	Erythromycin estolate
	Oral contraceptive	Norethynodrel with mestranol
	Oral hypoglycemic	Chlorpropamide
	Tranquilizer	Chlorpromazine*
Fatty liver	Chemotherapeutic	Tetracycline
	Anticonvulsant	Valproic acid (sodium valproate)
Hepatitis	Anesthetic	Halothane†
	Anticonvulsant	Phenytoin
	Antihypertensive	Methyldopa†
	Chemotherapeutic	Isoniazid†
	Diuretic	Chlorothiazide
	Laxative	Oxyphenisatin†
Toxic (necrosis)	Hydrocarbon	Carbon tetrachloride
	Metal	Yellow phosphorus
	Mushroom	Amanita phalloides
	Analgesic	Acetaminophen
Granulomas	Anti-inflammatory	Phenylbutazone
	Chemotherapeutic	Sulfonamides
	Xanthine inhibitor	Allopurinol

* Rarely associated with primary biliary cirrhosis-like lesion
† Occasionally associated with chronic active hepatitis or bridging hepatic necrosis and cirrhosis

Adapted from: Dienstag FL, Wands JR. In Braunwald E, Isselbacher KJ, Petersdorf RG, Wilson JD, Martin J, Fauci AS, editors: *Harrison's principles of internal medicine*, ed 11. New York, 1987, McGraw-Hill, p. 1336.

III-36 CAUSES OF PANCREATIC EXOCRINE INSUFFICIENCY

I. Alcohol, chronic alcoholism
II. Cystic fibrosis
III. Severe protein calorie malnutrition with hypoalbuminemia
IV. Pancreatic and duodenal neoplasms
V. Pancreatic resection
VI. Gastric surgery
   A. Subtotal gastrectomy with Billroth II anastomosis
   B. Subtotal gastrectomy with Billroth I anastomosis
   C. Truncal vagotomy with pyloroplasty
VII. Gastrinoma (Zollinger-Ellison syndrome)
VIII. Hereditary pancreatitis
IX. Traumatic pancreatitis
X. Hemochromatosis
XI. Shwachman's syndrome (pancreatic insufficiency and bone marrow dysfunction)
XII. Trypsinogen deficiency
XIII. Enterokinase deficiency
XIV. Radiation-induced chronic pancreatitis
XV. Alpha$_1$-antitrypsin deficiency
XVI. Idiopathic pancreatitis

Adapted from: Greenberger NJ, Isselbacher KJ, Toskes PP. In Braunwald E, Isselbacher KJ, Petersdorf RG, Wilson JD, Martin J, Fauci AS, editors: *Harrison's principles of internal medicine*, ed 11. New York, 1987, McGraw-Hill, p. 1378.

III-37 CAUSES OF ACUTE PANCREATITIS*

I. Alcohol ingestion (acute and chronic alcoholism)
II. Biliary tract disease (gallstones)
III. Postoperative (abdominal, nonabdominal)
IV. Postendoscopic retrograde cholangiopancreatography (ERCP)
V. Trauma (especially blunt abdominal trauma)
VI. Metabolic
   A. Hypertriglyceridemia
   B. Hyperparathyroidism
   C. Acute fatty liver of pregnancy
VII. Hereditary pancreatitis
VIII. Infections
   A. Mumps
   B. Viral hepatitis
   C. Mycoplasma
   D. Other viral infections (coxsackie and ECHO virus)
IX. Connective tissue disorders with vasculitis
   A. Systemic lupus erythematosus
   B. Necrotizing angiitis

III-37 CAUSES OF ACUTE PANCREATITIS*
(CONTINUED)

    C. Thrombotic thrombocytopenic purpura
    D. Henoch-Schönlein purpura
  X. Drug associated
    A. Definite association
       1. Azathioprine, 6-MP
       2. Sulfonamides
       3. Thiazide diuretics
       4. Furosemide
       5. Estrogens (oral contraceptives)
       6. Tetracycline
       7. Valproic acid
       8. DDI
       9. Pentamidine
      10. ACE inhibitors
    B. Probable association
       1. Chlorthalidone
       2. Ethacrynic acid
       3. Procainamide
       4. L-asparaginase
       5. Erythromycin
       6. Methyldopa
       7. Metronidazole
       8. NSAID's
    C. Equivocal association
       1. Corticosteroids
  XI. Obstruction of the ampulla of Vater
    A. Regional enteritis
    B. Duodenal diverticulum
 XII. Penetrating duodenal ulcer
XIII. Pancreas divisum
XIV. Recurrent bouts of acute pancreatitis without obvious cause
    A. Consider
       1. Occult disease of the gallbladder, biliary tree, pancreas, pancreatic ducts
       2. Drugs
       3. Hypertriglyceridemia
       4. Pancreas divisum
       5. Hereditary pancreatitis
       6. Pancreatic cancer
       7. Sphincter of Oddi dysfunction

*Modified from: Greenberger NJ, Toskes P, Isselbacher KJ. Diseases of the Pancreas. In Braunwald E, Isselbacher KJ, Petersdorf RG, Wilson JD, Martin J, Fauci AS, editors: *Harrison's principles of internal medicine*, ed 11. New York, 1987, McGraw-Hill.

III-38 FACTORS ADVERSELY INFLUENCING SURVIVAL IN ACUTE PANCREATITIS*

I. Risk factors indentifiable upon admission to hospital
  A. Increasing age
  B. Hypotension
  C. Tachycardia
  D. Abnormal physical examination of the lungs
  E. Abdominal mass
  F. Fever
  G. Leukocytosis
  H. Hyperglycemia
  I. First attack of pancreatitis

II. Risk factors identifiable during initial 48 hr of hospitalization
  A. Fall in hematocrit > 10% with hydration and/or hematocrit <30%
  B. Necessity for massive fluid and colloid replacement
  C. Hypocalcemia
  D. Hypoxemia with or without adult respiratory distress syndrome
  E. Hypoalbuminemia
  F. Azotemia

III. Major risk factors†
  A. Hypotension
  B. Need for massive fluid and colloid replacement
  C. Respiratory failure
  D. Hypocalcemia
  E. Hemorrhagic peritoneal fluid

IV. Apache score > 13

*Increased mortality can be expected if 3 or more risk factors in Groups I and II are present
†If 3 or more major risk factors from Group III are present, mortality rates can exceed 30%

Adapted from: Dienstag FL, Wands JR. In Braunwald E, Isselbacher KJ, Petersdorf RG, Wilson JD, Martin J, Fauci AS, editors: *Harrison's principles of internal medicine*, ed 11. New York, 1987, McGraw-Hill, p. 1336.

III-39 COMPLICATIONS OF ACUTE PANCREATITIS

I. Local
   A. Pancreatic phlegmon
   B. Pancreatic pseudocyst
      1. Pain
      2. Rupture with/without hemorrhage
      3. Hemorrhage
      4. Infection
   C. Pancreatic ascites
      1. Disruption of main pancreatic duct
      2. Leaking pseudocyst
   D. Pancreatic abscess
   E. Involvement of contiguous organs by necrotizing pancreatitis
      1. Massive intraperitoneal hemorrhage
      2. Thrombosis of blood vessels
      3. Bowel infarction
   F. Obstructive jaundice

II. Systemic
   A. Pulmonary
      1. Atelectasis
      2. Pneumonitis
      3. Pleural effusion
      4. Mediastinal abscess
      5. Adult respiratory distress syndrome
   B. Cardiovascular
      1. Hypotension
         a. hypovolemia
         b. hypoalbuminemia
      2. Sudden death
      3. Nonspecific ST-T changes in electrocardiogram simulating myocardial infarction
      4. Pericardial effusion
   C. Hematologic
      1. Disseminated intravascular coagulation (DIC)
   D. Gastrointestinal hemorrhage
      1. Peptic ulcer disease
      2. Erosive gastritis
      3. Hemorrhagic pancreatic necrosis with erosion into major blood vessels
      4. Portal vein thrombosis; variceal hemorrhage
   E. Renal
      1. Oliguria   } usually due to hypovolemia
      2. Azotemia
      3. Renal artery and/or renal vein thrombosis

III-39 COMPLICATIONS OF ACUTE PANCREATITIS (CONTINUED)

    F. Metabolic
        1. Hyperglycemia
        2. Hypertriglyceridemia
        3. Hypocalcemia
    G. Central nervous system
        1. Psychosis
        2. Fat emboli
        3. Encephalopathy
    H. Fat necrosis
        1. Subcutaneous tissues/erythematous nodules
        2. Bone
        3. Other organs (mediastinum, pleura, nervous system)
    I. Miscellaneous
        1. Sudden blindness (Purtscher's retinopathy)

Adapted from: Greenberger MJ, Toskes PP, Isselbacher KJ. In Braunwald E, Isselbacher KJ, Petersdorf RG, Wilson JD, Martin J, Fauci AS, editors: *Harrison's principles of internal medicine*, ed 11. New York, 1987, McGraw-Hill.

III-40 COMPLICATIONS OF CHRONIC PANCREATITIS

    I. Exocrine pancreatic insufficiency, steatorrhea, creatorrhea
   II. Vitamin B_{12} malabsorption
  III. Diabetes mellitus (difficult to exclude genetic diabetes)
  IV. Recurrent bouts of acute pancreatitis
   V. Pleural effusion (usually left-sided)
  VI. Pericardial effusion (rare)
 VII. Pancreatic ascites
    A. Disruption of pancreatic duct
    B. Leaking pseudocyst
VIII. Altered mental status (psychosis, etc.)
  IX. Ischemic necrosis of bone and intramedullary calcification
   X. Common bile duct stenosis, obstructive jaundice, biliary cirrhosis
  XI. Addiction to narcotics and analgesics
 XII. ? Increased incidence of pancreatic carcinoma (no firm evidence for this)
XIII. Non-diabetic retinopathy

III-41 DIAGNOSIS OF EXOCRINE PANCRE-ATIC INSUFFICIENCY (EPI)

I. Identify etiology of EPI
II. Steatorrhea* with/without creatorrhea; ↑ stool N_2
III. Pancreatic calcification*
IV. Diabetes mellitus*
V. Test of pancreatic exocrine function†
   A. Secretin with/without CCK-PZ → ↓ volume [HCO_3], ↓ enzyme output
   B. Tripeptide test (Bentiromide) → ↓ urine excretion of Para-aminobenzoic acid (PABA)
   C. Other indirect pancreatic function tests
   D. ↓ serum trypsinogen, ↓ serum pancreatic isoamylase
VI. ↓ Absorption of vitamin B_{12}
VII. Normal tests of mucosal function (D-xylose, small bowel mucosal biopsy)
VIII. Response to pancreatic enzyme therapy
   A. Weight gain
   B. ↓ steatorrhea, creatorrhea

*classical diagnostic triad
†frequently necessary as only 1/4 patients with exocrine pancreatic insufficiency have the classical diagnostic triad

III-42 POSTCHOLECYSTECTOMY SYNDROME

I. Definition: Persistence of abdominal pain after cholecystectomy
II. Causes
   A. Original diagnosis of cholecystitis/cholelithiasis as explanation for pain is incorrect
   B. Cholecystectomy not done, rather cholecystostomy performed
   C. Choledocholithiasis
      1. Stones missed at time of cholecystectomy
      2. Stones formed after cholecystectomy
   D. Common bile duct injury (stricture, etc.)
   E. Sclerosing cholangitis
   F. Bile duct carcinoma
   G. Chronic pancreatitis
   H. Sphincter of Oddi dysfunction
   I. Stenosis of papilla of Vater
   J. Anterior abdominal wall pain
      1. Scar tissue, traumatic neuroma, etc.

III-43 CRITERIA FOR ASSESSING SEVERITY OF MALNUTRITION

I. Anthropometric measurements
   A. Actual weight; ideal weight (↓ < 70% with severe malnutrition)
   B. Triceps skin fold thickness (reflects fat stores, severe depletion < 60%)
      1. Males — 12.5 mm
      2. Females — 16.5 mm
   C. Midarm muscle circumference (reflects protein stores, severe depletion < 60%)
      1. Males — 25.3 cm
      2. Females — 23.2 cm
II. Laboratory measurements
   A. Urinary creatinine (mg/24 hr): height (cm)
      1. Males — normal > 10.5
      2. Females — > 5.8
   B. Serum albumin < 3.0 gm/dl
   C. Serum transferrin < 150 µg/dl
   D. Absolute lymphocyte count < 800/ml

III-44 DIFFERENTIAL DIAGNOSIS OF HYPOALBUMINEMIA

I. Chronic renal disease with nephrotic syndrome
II. Chronic parenchymal liver disease
III. Malabsorption
IV. Malnutrition
V. Protein-losing enteropathy
VI. Burns
VII. Eczematoid dermatitis (severe)
VIII. Analbuminemia (failure to synthesize albumin)

III-45 GRANULOMATOUS LIVER DISEASE

I. Infections
  A. Viral (cytomegalovirus, Epstein-Barr virus)
  B. Bacterial (Brucella, Q fever, Mycobacterium)
  C. Fungal (histoplasmosis, coccidiomycosis, cryptococcosis, candidiasis, aspergillosis)
  D. Parasites (ascariasis, schistosomiasis, amebiasis)
  E. Spirochetes (syphilis)

II. Drug induced
  A. Sulfonamides
  B. Procainamide
  C. Phenytoin
  D. Allopurinol
  E. Phenylbutazone
  F. Isoniazid
  G. Methyldopa
  H. Quinidine
  I. Halothane
  J. Carbamazepine

III. Neoplasms
  A. Hodgkin's disease
  B. Non-Hodgkin's lymphoma

IV. Miscellaneous
  A. Sarcoidosis
  B. Primary biliary cirrhosis
  C. Regional enteritis
  D. Berylliosis

III-46 DELTA AGENT

I. General considerations
   A. Delta agent is a unique RNA virus which requires hepatitis B virus for its expression
   B. Delta infection has been transmitted to chimpanzees previously infected with hepatitis B virus
   C. Delta antibody has been measured in patients and is a reliable marker of Delta infection

II. Clinical aspects
   A. Delta agent + HBV infection (co-infection) usually results in an illness not different from classical hepatitis B
   B. Occasionally, co-infection can result in fulminant hepatitis
   C. Incidence of (+) Delta markers 20-50% in fulminant hepatitis
   D. Delta infection can aggravate pre-existing HBV liver disease or cause new disease in asymptomatic HB_sAg carriers
   E. Yucpa Indians — 18% fulminant hepatitis with Delta infection; high HB_sAg carriage rate
   F. High incidence of Delta agent (60-80%) in patients with chronic HBV liver disease
   G. What determines fulminant or chronic cause of Delta hepatitis?
      1. Active HBV infection with HB_eAg associated with severe acute illness
      2. Inactive HBV infection with HB_eAg associated with chronicity
   H. Chronic hepatitis in 137 hepatitis B carriers and intrahepatic Delta antigen
      1. Fatal outcome in 12.8% with F/U 2-6 years
      2. 31/75 patients (41%) developed manifest cirrhosis in 2-6 years F/U

Conclusion: Chronic delta infection worsens the histologic lesion and accelerates the course of liver disease.

Reference: Greenberger NJ. *Gastrointestinal disorders: a pathophysiological approach*, ed 4. Chicago, 1989, Year Book Medical Publishers, p. 321.

III-47 PRIMARY SCLEROSING CHOLANGITIS

   I. Definition:
     A. Obliterative inflammatory fibrosis of the extrahepatic bile ducts with or without intrahepatic duct involvement

  II. Histologic features:
     A. ↓ Number of bile ducts
     B. Ductular proliferation
     C. Portal inflammation
     D. Substantial copper deposition
     E. Piecemeal necrosis
     F. Cirrhosis

 III. Diseases associated with PSC
     A. Idiopathic ulcerative colitis (UC)   (50% to 75%)
     B. Granulomatous colitis/ileocolitis   (< 5%)
     C. Thyroiditis   (< 5%)
     D. Pancreatitis   (< 5%)
     E. Sicca syndrome   (< 5%)
     F. Hypothyroidism   (< 5%)

 IV. Clinical features
     A. 70% are males
     B. Presenting features
       1. Jaundice
       2. Pruritus
       3. Abdominal pain
       4. Hepatosplenomegaly
       5. Abnormal liver tests
     C. May precede or follow IUC
     D. Mean survival ~ 5 years
     E. Death usually due to liver failure
     F. Copper overload ≃ PBC
     G. Screen for PSC in IUC patients with ↑ Alk. Phos.

PSC = primary sclerosing cholangitis
PBC = primary biliary cirrhosis
IUC = idiopathic ulcerative colitis

Reference: Greenberger NJ. *Gastrointestinal disorders: a pathophysiological approach*, ed 4. Chicago, 1989, Year Book Medical Publishers, p. 418.

III-48 PREDISPOSING FACTORS FOR CHOLESTEROL AND PIGMENT GALLSTONE FORMATION

I. Cholesterol and mixed stones
   A. Demography
      1. Northern Europe and North and South America greater than Orient; probable familial, hereditary aspects
   B. Obesity
      1. Normal bile acid secretion but ↑ biliary secretion of cholesterol
   C. Weight loss
      1. ↑ biliary cholesterol secretion while ↓ enteropathic secretion of bile salt
   D. Female sex hormones
      1. Estrogens stimulate ↑ liver uptake of dietary cholesterol, and ↑ biliary cholesterol.
      2. Oral contraceptives ↓ bile acid pool size and bile salt secretions
   E. Ileal disease or resection
      1. Malabsorption of bile acids leads to ↓ bile acid pool and ↓ biliary secretion of bile salts
   F. Increasing age
      1. ↑ biliary secretion of cholesterol, ↓ size of bile acid pool, ↓ biliary secretion of bile salts.
   G. Gallbladder hypomotility leading to stasis and formation sludge
      1. Prolonged parenteral nutrition
      2. Fasting
      3. Pregnancy
      4. Drugs such as octreotide
   H. Clofibrate therapy
      1. ↑ biliary secretion of cholesterol
II. Pigment stones
   A. Demographic/genetic factors: orient, rural setting
   B. Chronic hemolysis
   C. Alcoholic cirrhosis
   D. Chronic biliary tract infection, parasite infestation
   E. Increasing age

III-49 CAUSES OF FULMINANT HEPATIC FAILURE

I. Infectious
   A. Common causes
      1. Viral hepatitis A, B, D, E
      2. Non-A, non-B (?C) hepatitis
   B. Rare causes
      1. Cytomegalovirus
      2. Epstein-Barr virus
      3. Herpes simplex virus
      4. Paramyxovirus (syncytial giant cell hepatitis)
II. Metabolic
   A. Acute fatty liver of pregnancy
   B. Reye's syndrome
III. Drugs/chemical exposure
   A. Carbon tetrachloride
   B. *Amanita phalloides* mushroom poisoning
   C. Acetaminophen overdose
   D. Tetracycline
   E. Halothane
   F. Sodium valproate
   G. Isoniazid
   H. Methyldopa
   I. Monoamine oxidase inhibitors
   J. Yellow phosphorus
   K. Nonsteroidal anti-inflammatory drugs
IV. Ischemic/hypoxic
   A. Hepatic arterial or venous occlusion
   B. Shock
   C. Hyperthermia
   D. Primary graft nonfunction post liver transplantation
V. Disorders presenting as fulminant hepatic failure with histological evidence of chronic liver disease
   A. Wilson's disease
   B. Massive malignant infiltration of the liver
   C. Liver failure postjejunoileal bypass
   D. Autoimmune chronic active hepatitis
   E. Chronic hepatitis B with reactivation or delta superinfection
   F. Erythropoietic protoporphyria

From Fingerote RJ, Bain VG. Fulminant hepatic failure. *Am. J. Gastro.* 88:1000, 1993.

CHAPTER IV
HEMATOLOGY—ONCOLOGY

IV-1 DIFFERENTIAL DIAGNOSIS OF NORMOCHROMIC-NORMOCYTIC ANEMIA

I. Primary bone marrow failure
   A. Aplastic anemia
   B. Myelophthisic anemia
      1. Leukemia and lymphoma
      2. Other neoplasms
      3. Myelofibrosis
      4. Granulomas
II. Secondary anemias
   A. Anemia of chronic inflammation
      1. Connective tissue disease
      2. Chronic infection
   B. Anemia of uremia
   C. Anemias associated with endocrinopathies
      1. Hypothyroidism
      2. Addison's disease
      3. Hypogonadism
      4. Panhypopituitarism
   D. Anemia associated with chronic liver disease
   E. Recent blood loss
   F. HIV infection
   G. Acute hemolysis

Modified from: Bunn HF. In Isselbacher KJ, Adams RD, Braunwald E, Petersdorf RG, Wilson JD, editors: *Harrison's principles of internal medicine,* ed 10. New York, 1983, McGraw-Hill p. 289.

IV-2 DIFFERENTIAL DIAGNOSIS OF MICROCYTIC-HYPOCHROMIC ANEMIA

I. Iron deficiency anemia
   A. Nutritional deficiency
   B. Chronic blood loss
   C. Gastric surgery and achlorhydria
   D. Improved absorption
   E. Increased requirements (e.g., pregnancy)
II. Sideroblastic anemia
   A. Hereditary or congenital
      1. X-linked
      2. Autosomal recessive
   B. Acquired sideroblastic anemia
      1. Idiopathic refractory sideroblastic anemia
      2. Secondary to underlying disease
         a. Neoplasms
         b. Inflammatory
         c. Hematologic
         d. Metabolic
      3. Associated with drugs or toxins
         a. Ethanol
         b. Lead
         c. Antituberculosis agents
         d. Chloramphenicol
         e. Alkylating agents
III. Thalassemia
IV. Chronic disease

Modified from: Lee GR, Wintrobe MM, Bunn FH. In Isselbacher KJ, Adams RD, Braunwald E, Petersdorf RG, Wilson JD, editors: *Harrison's principles of internal medicine,* ed 9. New York, 1980, pp. 1515, 1517.

IV-3 DIFFERENTIAL DIAGNOSIS OF MACROCYTIC ANEMIAS

I. Vitamin B$_{12}$ deficiency
   A. Inadequate intake (rare)
   B. Malabsorption
      1. Low intrinsic factor
         a. Pernicious anemia
         b. Postgastrectomy
         c. Congenital absence of intrinsic factor
      2. Disorders of terminal ileum
         a. Surgical resection
         b. Sprue
         c. Inflammatory bowel disease
         d. Neoplasms

3. Competition for vitamin B_{12}
   a. Fish tapeworm
   b. Bacteria: blind loop syndrome
4. Drugs
   a. *p*-aminosalicylic acid
   b. Colchicine
   c. Neomycin
C. Transcobalamin II deficiency
II. Folate deficiency
  A. Inadequate intake
  B. Malabsorption
     1. Sprue
     2. Drugs (phenytoin, barbiturates)
  C. Increased requirements
     1. Pregnancy
     2. Infancy
     3. Malignancy
     4. Chronic hemolytic anemia
     5. Chronic exfoliative dermatitis
     6. Hemodialysis
  D. Impaired metabolism
     1. Drugs that inhibit dihydrofolate reductase
        (methotrexate, pentamidine, triamterene)
     2. Alcohol
     3. Enzyme deficiencies
III. Myelodysplastic syndromes
IV. Miscellaneous
  A. Chemotherapeutic agents which interfere with DNA
     metabolism
     1. 6-Mercaptopurine
     2. Azathioprine
     3. 5-Fluorouracil
     4. Cytosine arabinoside
     5. Procarbazine
     6. Hydroxyurea
     7. Acyclovir
     8. Zidovudine
  B. Spherocytosis
  C. Hypothyroidism
  D. Liver disease
  E. Reticulocytosis
  F. Hereditary orotic aciduria and other rare metabolic
     disorders
  G. Di Guglielmo's syndrome (acute erythroleukemia)

IV-3 DIFFERENTIAL DIAGNOSIS OF MACROCYTIC ANEMIAS (CONTINUED)

Modified from: Babior BM, Bunn HF. In Braunwald E, Isselbacher KJ, Petersdorf RG, Wilson JD, Martin J, Fauci AS, Root RK, editors: *Harrison's principles of internal medicine*, ed 12. New York, 1991, McGraw-Hill, p. 1523.

IV-4 DIFFERENTIAL DIAGNOSIS OF HEMOLYTIC ANEMIAS

I. Inherited disorders
   A. Defects in the erythrocyte membrane
      1. Hereditary spherocytosis
      2. Hereditary elliptocytosis
      3. Abetalipoproteinemia
      4. Hereditary stomatocytosis
      5. LCAT deficiency
   B. Deficiency of erythrocyte glycolytic enzymes
      1. Pyruvate kinase
      2. Hexokinase
      3. Aldolase
   C. Abnormalities of erythrocyte nucleotide metabolism
      1. Pyrimidine 5'nucleotidase deficiency
      2. Adenosine deaminase excess
      3. Adenosine triphosphatase deficiency
      4. Adenylate kinase deficiency
   D. Deficiencies of enzymes involved in the pentose phosphate pathway and in glutathione metabolism
      1. G-6-PD
      2. Glutamyl-cysteine synthetase
      3. Glutathione synthetase
      4. Glutathione reductase
   E. Defects in globin structure and synthesis
      1. Sickle cell anemia
      2. Thalassemia major
      3. Hemoglobin H disease
II. Acquired disorders
   A. Immunohemolytic anemias
      1. Secondary to transfusion of incompatible blood
      2. Hemolytic disease of the newborn
      3. Due to warm reactive antibodies
         a. Idiopathic
         b. "Secondary"
            (1) Virus and mycoplasma infection
            (2) Lymphosarcoma and CLL

IV-4 DIFFERENTIAL DIAGNOSIS OF HEMOLYTIC ANEMIAS (CONTINUED)

        (3) Other malignancies
        (4) Immune-deficiency states
        (5) Systemic lupus erythematosus and other
            "autoimmune" disorders
        (6) Drug induced
    4. Due to cold reactive antibodies
        a. Cold hemagglutinin disease
        b. Paroxysmal cold hemoglobinuria
  B. Traumatic and microangiopathic hemolytic anemias
    1. Prosthetic valves and other cardiac abnormalities
    2. Hemolytic-uremic syndrome
    3. Thrombotic thrombocytopenic purpura
    4. Disseminated intravascular coagulation
    5. Graft rejection
    6. Immune complex disease
  C. Infectious agents
    1. Protozoan
        a. Malaria
        b. Toxoplasmosis
        c. Leishmaniasis
        d. Trypanosomiasis
    2. Bacterial
        a. Bartonellosis
        b. Clostridial infections
        c. Typhoid fever
        d. Cholera
  D. Chemicals, drugs and venoms
    1. Oxidant drugs and chemicals
        a. Naphthalene
        b. Nitrofurantoin
        c. Sulfonamides
    2. Non-oxidant chemicals
        a. Arsine
        b. Copper
        c. Water
    3. Associated with hemodialysis and uremia
    4. Venoms
  E. Physical agents
    1. Thermal injury
  F. Hypophosphatemia
  G. "Spur cell" anemia in liver disease
  H. Paroxysmal nocturnal hemoglobinuria
  I. Vitamin E deficiency in newborns

Modified from: Wintrobe, et al. In *Clinical hematology*, ed 9, vol 1.
Philadelphia, 1993, Lea & Febiger, p. 94

IV-5 DIFFERENTIAL DIAGNOSIS OF PANCYTOPENIA

I. Aplastic anemia
II. Pancytopenia with normal or increased bone marrow cellularity
  A. Myelodysplastic syndromes
  B. Hypersplenism
  C. Vitamin B_{12} or folate deficiency
III. Bone marrow replacement
  A. Hematologic malignancies
  B. Nonhematologic metastatic tumor
  C. Storage-cell disorders
  D. Osteopetrosis
  E. Myelofibrosis
IV. Paroxysmal nocturnal hemoglobinuria
V. Infections
  A. HIV
  B. Tuberculosis
  C. Atypical mycobacterium
  D. Fungal
  E. Cytomegalovirus

Adapted from: Rappeport JM, Bunn HF. In Braunwald E, Isselbacher KJ, Petersdorf RG, Wilson JD, Martin J, Fauci AS, Root RK, editors: *Harrison's principles of internal medicine*, ed 12. New York, 1991, McGraw-Hill, p. 1568.

IV-6 DIFFERENTIAL DIAGNOSIS OF APLASTIC ANEMIA

I. Idiopathic
II. Constitutional (Fanconi's anemia, also called Fanconi's syndrome)
III. Chemical and physical agents
   A. Dose-related
      1. Chloramphenicol
      2. Benzene
      3. Ionizing irradiation
      4. Alkylating agents
      5. Antimetabolites (folic acid antagonists, purine and pyrimidine analogues)
      6. Mitotic inhibitors
      7. Anthracyclines
      8. Inorganic arsenicals
   B. Idiosyncratic
      1. Acetazolamide
      2. Arsenicals
      3. Barbiturates
      4. Chloramphenicol
      5. Gold
      6. Insecticides
      7. Phenothiazines
      8. Phenylbutazone
      9. Pyrimethamine
      10. Solvents
      11. Sulfa drugs
      12. Thiouracils
IV. Viral Infections
   A. Hepatitis (esp. HCV)
   B. Epstein-Barr
   C. Parvovirus
   D. HIV
   E. Cytomegalovirus
V. Immunologically mediated aplasia
VI. Pregnancy
VII. Paroxysmal nocturnal hemoglobinuria
VIII. Miscellaneous: Systemic lupus erythematosus, pancreatitis, miliary tuberculosis, Simmonds' disease, viral infections

Adapted from: Rappeport JM, Bunn HF. In Braunwald E, Isselbacher KJ, Petersdorf RG, Wilson JD, Martin J, Fauci AS, Root RK, editors: *Harrison's principles of internal medicine*, ed 12. New York, 1991, McGraw-Hill, p. 1568.

IV-7 DIFFERENTIAL DIAGNOSIS OF NEUTROPENIA

I. Decreased production
   A. Hematologic diseases
      1. Aplastic anemia
      2. Cyclic neutropenia
      3. Leukemia
      4. Chediak-Higashi Syndrome
      5. Myelodysplastic syndromes
      6. Chronic idiopathic neutropenia
   B. Drug-induced condition
      1. Agranulocytosis
      2. Myelotoxic drugs
   C. Malignancies with marrow invasion
   D. Nutritional deficiencies
      1. Vitamin B_{12}
      2. Folate
      3. Copper
   E. Infections
      1. Tuberculosis
      2. Typhoid
      3. Mononucleosis
      4. Malaria
      5. Brucellosis
      6. Tularemia
      7. Measles
      8. Viral hepatitis
      9. Histoplasmosis
      10. HIV
II. Peripheral destruction
   A. Autoimmune disorders
      1. Felty's syndrome
      2. Systemic lupus erythematosus
   B. Splenic trapping
   C. Antineutrophil antibodies
III. Peripheral margination
   A. Overwhelming bacterial infection
   B. Hemodialysis
   C. Cardiopulmonary bypass

Modified from: Dale DC. In Braunwald E, Isselbacher KJ, Petersdorf RG, Wilson JD, Martin J, Fauci AS, Root RK, editors: *Harrison's principles of internal medicine*, ed 12. New York, 1991, McGraw-Hill, p. 361.

IV-8 DIFFERENTIAL DIAGNOSIS OF NEUTROPHILIA

I. Physiologic
  A. Exercise
  B. Epinephrine
  C. Pain, emotion, or stress
II. Infections
  A. Bacterial
  B. Parasitic
  C. Fungal
  D. Viral (less common)
III. Inflammation
  A. Burns
  B. Tissue necrosis
    1. Myocardial infarction
    2. Pulmonary infarction
  C. Connective tissue disease
  D. Other inflammatory diseases
IV. Metabolic disorders
  A. Diabetic ketoacidosis
  B. Acute renal failure
  C. Eclampsia
  D. Poisoning
V. Myeloproliferative diseases
VI. Miscellaneous
  A. Metastatic carcinoma
  B. Acute hemorrhage or hemolysis
  C. Glucocorticosteroids
  D. Lithium therapy
  E. Idiopathic

Modified from: Dale DC. In Braunwald E, Isselbacher KJ, Petersdorf RG, Wilson JD, Martin J, Fauci AS, Root RK, editors: *Harrison's principles of internal medicine*, ed 12. New York, 1991, McGraw-Hill, p. 360.

IV-9 DIFFERENTIAL DIAGNOSIS OF EOSINOPHILIA

I. Allergic disorders
   A. Hay fever
   B. Asthma
   C. Urticaria
II. Drug reactions
   A. Iodine
   B. Aspirin
   C. Cephalosporins
   D. Sulfonamides
III. Dermatologic disorders including:
   A. Pemphigus
   B. Dermatitis herpetiformis
IV. Parasitic infections
   A. Trichinosis
   B. Echinococcus
   C. Strongyloides
V. Pulmonary infiltrate with eosinophilia
VI. Malignancy
   A. Hodgkin's disease
   B. Chronic myelogenous leukemia
   C. Mycosis fungoides
   D. Carcinoma of lung, stomach, pancreas, ovary, or uterus
VII. Connective tissue disease
   A. Rheumatoid arthritis
   B. Dermatomyositis
   C. Periarteritis nodosa
   D. Vasculitis syndrome (leukocytoclastic, hypersensitivity)
VIII. Hypereosinophilic syndromes
   A. Loeffler's endocarditis
   B. Eosinophilic leukemia
IX. Chronic granulomatosis disease (sarcoidosis)
X. Miscellaneous
   A. Adrenal insufficiency
XI. Idiopathic

Modified from: Dale DC. In Braunwald E, Isselbacher KJ, Petersdorf RG, Wilson JD, Martin J, Fauci AS, Root RK, editors: *Harrison's principles of internal medicine*, ed 12. New York, 1991, McGraw-Hill, p. 362.

IV-10 DIFFERENTIAL DIAGNOSIS OF BASOPHILIA

I. Hematologic disorders
   A. Hodgkin's disease
   B. Myeloproliferative diseases
      1. Chronic myelogenous leukemia
      2. Polycythemia vera
   C. Carcinoma
   D. Myelofibrosis
   E. Basophilic leukemia
II. Chronic inflammatory conditions
   A. Ulcerative colitis
   B. Chronic sinusitis
   C. Occasionally with nephrosis
III. Myxedema
IV. Infections
   A. Influenza
   B. Varicella
   C. Tuberculosis
V. Miscellaneous
   A. Mastocytosis
   B. Estrogen administration
   C. Drug hypersensitivity
   D. Radiation exposure

Modified from: Wintrobe MM, et al., editors. In *Clinical hematology*, ed 8, vol 1. Philadelphia, 1981, Lea & Febiger, pp. 1300-1301.

IV-11 DISORDERS ASSOCIATED WITH MONOCYTOSIS

I. Hematologic disorders
   - A. Hemopoietic stem cell disorders
      1. Preleukemia
      2. Acute myelogenous leukemia
      3. Chronic myelogenous leukemia
      4. Polycythemia vera
   - B. Lymphocytic tumors
      1. Lymphoma
      2. Multiple myeloma
   - C. Histiocytosis
   - D. Hemolytic anemia
   - E. ITP
   - F. Chronic neutropenias
   - G. Postsplenectomy
II. Inflammatory and immune disorders
   - A. Collagen diseases
   - B. Gastrointestinal disorders
      1. Ulcerative colitis
      2. Regional enteritis
      3. Sprue
      4. Alcoholic liver disease
   - C. Sarcoidosis
   - D. Infections
III. Miscellaneous conditions
   - A. Hand-Schüller-Christian disease
   - B. Glucocorticoids
   - C. Parturition

Modified from: Lichtman R. In Williams WJ, Beutler E, Erslev AJ, Lichtman MA, editors: *Hematology*, ed 4. New York, 1990, McGraw-Hill, p. 883

IV-12 DIFFERENTIAL DIAGNOSIS OF ABNORMALITIES FOUND ON PERIPHERAL SMEAR

I. Basophilic stippling
   - A. Lead poisoning
   - B. Heavy metal poisoning
   - C. Severe anemia
II. Howell-Jolly bodies
   - A. Severe hemolytic anemia
   - B. Pernicious anemia
   - C. Leukemia
   - D. Thalassemia
   - E. Postsplenectomy

IV-12 DIFFERENTIAL DIAGNOSIS OF ABNORMALITIES FOUND ON PERIPHERAL SMEAR (CONTINUED)

III. Pappenheimer bodies
   A. Thalassemia
   B. Lead poisoning
   C. Di Guglielmo's syndrome
IV. Heinz-Ehrlich bodies
   A. Glucose-6-PD deficiency
   B. Drug-induced hemolytic anemias
V. Spherocytes
   A. Autoimmune hemolytic anemia
   B. Congenital spherocytosis
VI. Stomatocytes
   A. Acute alcohol (transient)
   B. Drugs (e.g., phenothiazines)
   C. Neoplastic, cardiovascular, hepatobiliary disease
   D. Hereditary
VII. Target cells
   A. Hemoglobin C disease or trait
   B. Thalassemia minor
   C. Iron deficiency anemia
   D. Liver disease
   E. Postsplenectomy
VIII. Ovalocytes
   A. Microcytic anemia
   B. Hereditary
   C. Megaloblastic anemias
IX. Teardrop
   A. Spent polycythemia vera
   B. Myelofibrosis
   C. Thalassemia (esp. homozygous b)
X. Sickle cells
XI. Acanthocytes
   A. Abetalipoproteinemia
   B. Postsplenectomy
   C. Fulminant liver disease
XII. Helmet
   A. DIC
   B. Severe valvular heart disease
   C. Prosthetic heart valves
   D. Microangiopathic hemolytic anemia
   E. Snake bite

Adapted from: Wallach J. In *Interpretation of diagnostic tests*, ed 4. Boston, 1986, Little, Brown, pp. 120-122.

IV-13 DIFFERENTIAL DIAGNOSIS OF ERYTHROCYTOSIS

I. Erythrocytosis associated with a normal or reduced red cell mass (spurious)
   A. Acute or chronic hemoconcentration (relative)
   B. Spurious polycythemia (also called stress polycythemia or Gaisböck's syndrome)
II. Erythrocytosis associated with an elevated red cell mass (absolute polycythemia)
   A. Polycythemia vera
   B. Secondary polycythemia (increased erythropoietin production)
      1. Systemic hypoxia
         a. High altitude
         b. Cardiac disease with right to left shunt
         c. Chronic pulmonary disease
      2. Decreased blood oxygen carrying capacity, increase in carboxyhemoglobin or methemoglobin
      3. Impaired oxygen delivery, hemoglobin with increased oxygen affinity or congenital decreased red cell 2,3-diphosphoglycerate
      4. Local hypoxia — renal artery stenosis
      5. Autonomous erythropoietin production
         a. Tumors
            (1) Hypernephroma
            (2) Cerebella hemangioblastoma
            (3) Hepatoma
            (4) Uterine fibroids
            (5) Pheochromocytoma
            (6) Adrenal cortical adenoma
            (7) Ovarian carcinoma
         b. Renal disorders
            (1) Cysts
            (2) Hydronephrosis
            (3) Bartter's syndrome
            (4) Transplantation
      6. Familial polycythemia due to autonomous erythropoietin production

Reference: Hoffman R, et al. In Stollerman GH, editor: *Advances in internal medicine*, vol 24. Chicago, 1979, Yearbook Medical Publishers, p. 260.

IV-14 CRITERIA FOR THE DIAGNOSIS OF POLYCYTHEMIA VERA

I. Major criteria
   A. Increased red cell mass
   B. Arterial O_2 saturation $\geq 92\%$
   C. Splenomegaly
II. Minor criteria
   A. Thrombocytosis
   B. Leukocytosis
   C. Elevated serum B_{12}
   D. Increased leukocyte alkaline phosphatase
   E. Increased serum B_{12} (> 900 pg/ml) or unbound B_{12} binding capacity (> 2,200 pg/ml)

Diagnosis of polycythemia vera is made if patient has all three major criteria *or* the first two major criteria and any two minor criteria

III. Most common presenting symptoms of patients in the national polycythemia vera study

Symptoms	Percentage
Headache	49
Weakness	47
Pruritus	46
Dizziness	45
Sweating	33
Weight loss	31
Paresthesias	29
Joint symptoms	28
Epigastric distress	28

Reference: Berlin NI. Diagnosis and classification of polycythemias. *Semin Hematol* 12:339, 1975.

IV-15 DIFFERENTIAL DIAGNOSIS OF THROMBOCYTOSIS

I. Myeloproliferative disorders
   A. Primary thrombocythemia
   B. Polycythemia vera
   C. Chronic myelogenous leukemia
   D. Agnogenic myeloid metaplasia
II. Chronic inflammatory disorders
   A. Rheumatoid arthritis
   B. Acute rheumatic fever
   C. Polyarteritis nodosa
   D. Wegener's granulomatosis
   E. Ulcerative colitis
   F. Regional enteritis
   G. Tuberculosis
   H. Hepatic cirrhosis
   I. Sarcoidosis
III. Acute hemorrhage
IV. Iron deficiency anemia
V. Hemolytic anemia
VI. Malignancy
VII. Post-splenectomy
VIII. Response to drugs
   A. Vincristine
   B. Epinephrine
IX. Response to exercise
X. Osteoporosis

Modified from Williams WJ. In Williams WJ, Beutler E, Erslev AJ, Lichtman MA, editors: *Hematology*, ed 4. New York, 1990, McGraw-Hill, p. 1403.

IV-16 MYELODYSPLASTIC SYNDROMES

I. Refractory anemia
II. Refractory anemia with ringed sideroblasts
III. Refractory anemia with excess blasts
IV. Refractory anemia with excess blasts in transformation
V. Chronic myelomonocytic leukemia

IV-17 MYELOPROLIFERATIVE SYNDROMES

I. Chronic myelogenous leukemia
II. Polycythemia rubra vera
III. Myelofibrosis
IV. Essential thrombocythemia

IV-18 STAGING OF CHRONIC LYMPHOCYTIC LEUKEMIA

I. RAI classification

0 Lymphocytosis > 15,000 mm³; marrow 40% lymphocytes
1 Lymphocytosis plus lymphadenopathy
2 Lymphocytosis plus hepato- or splenomegaly
3 Lymphocytosis plus anemia
4 Lymphocytosis plus thrombocytopenia

II. Median survival of RAI classes

0 > 150 months
1 105 months
2 71 months
3 19 months
4 19 months

Modified from: Rai, et al. *Blood* 46:219, 1975

IV-19 CRITERIA FOR THE DIAGNOSIS OF MULTIPLE MYELOMA

I. Major criteria
  A. Plasmacytoma
  B. IgG paraprotein > 3.5 gm%
     IgA paraprotein > 2 gm%
     Light chain in urine > 1 gm%
  C. Bone marrow plasma cells > 30%
II. Minor criteria
  A. Bone marrow plasma cells 10-30%
  B. IgG paraprotein < 3.5 gm%
         IgA paraprotein < 2 gm%
  C. Lytic bone lesions
  D. Hypogammaglobulinemia (IgA < 100 mg/dl, IgM < 50 mg/dl)
III. To make the diagnosis (one of the following)
  A. A +B, C, or D from II above
  B. B + B, C, or D from II above
  C. C from II above
  D. A + B + C or A + B + D from II above

Adapted from: Southwest Oncology Group Protocol, 7927

IV-20 STAGING SYSTEM FOR MULTIPLE MYELOMA

Stage	Criteria	Measured myeloma cell mass (cells on $10^{12}/m^2$)
I	All of the following Hemoglobin value >10 g/dl Serum calcium value > 12 mg/dl On x-ray; normal bone structure (scale 0) or solitary osseous myeloma Low M component level IgG < 5 g/dl IgA < 3 g/dl Urine light chain M component < 4 g/24h	< 0.6 (low)
II	Fitting between stage I and stage III	0.6-1.2 (intermediate)
III	One or more of the following Hemoglobin value < 8.5 g/dl Serum calcium value > 12 mg/dl Advanced lytic bone lesions (scale 3) High M component level IgG > 7 g/dl IgA > 5 g/dl Urine light chain M component > 12 g/24h	$\geq$ 1.2 (high)

Subclassification
A: Relatively normal renal function (serum creatinine value < 2 mg/dl)
B: Abnormal renal function (serum creatinine value > 2 mg/dl)

Reference: Jandi J. In: *Blood: textbook of hematology.* Boston, 1987, Little, Brown, p. 831.

IV-21 RENAL AND ELECTROLYTE DISORDERS IN MULTIPLE MYELOMA

I. "Myeloma kidney"
II. Renal tubular dysfunction
III. Acute renal failure
IV. Amyloidosis
V. Plasma cell invasion of the kidneys
VI. Hypercalcemia
VII. Hyperuricemia
VIII. Spurious hyponatremia
IX. Urinary tract infections

Reference: Fer MF, et al. *Am J Med* 71:707, 1981.

IV-22 CRITERIA FOR THE DIAGNOSIS OF THROMBOTIC THROMBOCYTOPENIC PURPURA

I. Fever
II. Microangiopathic hemolytic anemia (Coombs negative)
III. Thrombocytopenia
IV. Neurologic disorders
V. Renal dysfunction

IV-23 DIFFERENTIAL DIAGNOSIS OF SPLENOMEGALY

I. Infections
   A. Mononucleosis
   B. Bacterial septicemia
   C. Tuberculosis
   D. Malaria
   E. Viral hepatitis
   F. AIDS
   G. Congenital syphilis
   H. Splenic abscess
   I. Disseminated histoplasmosis

II. Disordered immunoregulation
   A. Rheumatoid arthritis (Felty's syndrome)
   B. Systemic lupus erythematosus
   C. Immune hemolytic anemia
   D. Angioimmunoblastic lymphadenopathy
   E. Drug reactions with serum sickness
   F. Immune thrombocytopenia and neutropenia

III. Altered splenic blood flow
   A. Laennec's and postnecrotic cirrhosis
   B. Hepatic vein obstruction
   C. Portal vein obstruction
   D. Congestive heart failure
   E. Splenic artery aneurysm

IV. Abnormal erythrocytes
   A. Spherocytosis
   B. Sickle cell disease
   C. Thalassemia

V. Infiltrative diseases
   A. Benign: amyloidosis, Gaucher's, Niemann-Pick, Hurlers, extramedullary hematopoiesis, splenic cysts.
   B. Malignant: leukemias, lymphomas, myeloproliferative syndromes, angiosarcoma, metastatic tumors.

VI. Miscellaneous
   A. Thyrotoxicosis
   B. Iron deficiency anemia
   C. Sarcoidosis
   D. Berylliosis

Modified from: Haynes B. In Braunwald E, Isselbacher KJ, Petersdorf RG, Wilson JD, Martin J, Fauci AS, Root RK, editors: *Harrison's principles of internal medicine*, ed 12. New York, 1991, McGraw-Hill, p. 357.

IV-24 DIFFERENTIAL DIAGNOSIS OF LYMPHADENOPATHY

I. Infectious diseases
  A. Viral
    1. HIV
    2. Mononucleosis
    3. Cytomegalovirus
    4. Infectious hepatitis
  B. Bacterial
    1. Pyogenic streptococcal or staphylococcal
    2. Brucellosis
  C. Fungal
    1. Histoplasmosis
    2. Cocciodiomycosis
  D. Mycobacterial
  E. Parasitic
    1. Toxoplasmosis
    2. Malaria
  F. Spirochetal
II. Immunologic diseases
  A. Rheumatoid arthritis
  B. Systemic lupus
  C. Dermatomyositis
  D. Serum sickness
  E. Drug reactions
  F. Angioimmunoblastic lymphadenopathy
III. Malignant diseases
  A. Hematologic
    1. Lymphoma
    2. Malignant histiocytosis
    3. Acute leukemia
    4. Myeloproliferative syndromes
    5. Chronic lymphocytic leukemia
  B. Metastatic tumors to lymph nodes
IV. Endocrine diseases: hyperthyroidism
V. Lipid storage diseases
  A. Gaucher's disease
  B. Niemann-Pick disease
VI. Miscellaneous
  A. Sinus histiocytosis
  B. Sarcoidosis
  C. Amyloidosis
  D. Lymphomatoid granulomatosis
  E. Mucocutaneous lymph node syndrome
  F. Giant (angiofollicular) lymph node hyperplasia
  G. Dermatopathic lymphadenitis

IV-24 DIFFERENTIAL DIAGNOSIS OF LYMPHADENOPATHY (CONTINUED)

Modified from: Haynes B. In Braunwald E, Isselbacher KJ, Petersdorf RG, Wilson JD, Martin J, Fauci AS, Root RK, editors: *Harrison's principles of internal medicine*, ed 12. New York, 1991, McGraw-Hill, p. 355.

IV-25 DIFFERENTIAL DIAGNOSIS OF THROMBOCYTOPENIA

  I. Decreased marrow production
    A. Marrow infiltration with tumor, fibrosis
    B. Marrow failure: aplastic and hypoplastic anemias
    C. ? HIV
  II. Splenic sequestration
    A. Splenic hypertrophy: tumor, portal hypertension
  III. Increased destruction
    A. Nonimmune
      1. Vascular prostheses, cardiac valves
      2. DIC
      3. Sepsis
      4. Vasculitis
      5. Thrombotic thrombocytopenia purpura
    B. Immune
      1. Autoantibodies to platelet antigens (e.g., ITP)
      2. Drug-associated antibodies
      3. Circulatory immune complexes: lupus, viral agents, bacterial sepsis
      4. HIV

Adapted from: Handin R. In Braunwald E, Isselbacher KJ, Petersdorf RG, Wilson JD, Martin J, Fauci AS, Root RK, editors: *Harrison's principles of internal medicine*, ed 12. New York, 1991, McGraw-Hill, p. 352.

IV-26 CAUSES OF CYANOSIS

I. Central cyanosis
  A. Decreased arterial oxygen saturation
    1. Decreased atmospheric pressure-high altitude
    2. Impaired pulmonary function
      a. Alveolar hypoventilation
      b. Pulmonary ventilation/perfusion mismatching
      c. Impaired oxygen diffusion
    3. Anatomic shunts
      a. Certain types of congenital heart disease
      b. Pulmonary arteriovenous fistulas
      c. Multiple small intrapulmonary shunts
    4. Hemoglobin with low affinity for oxygen
  B. Hemoglobin abnormalities
    1. Methemoglobinemia-hereditary, acquired
    2. Sulfhemoglobinemia-acquired
    3. Carboxyhemoglobinemia (not true cyanosis)
II. Peripheral cyanosis
  A. Reduced cardiac output
  B. Cold exposure
  C. Redistribution of blood flow from extremities
  D. Arterial obstruction
  E. Venous obstruction

Modified from: Braunwald E. In Braunwald E, Isselbacher KJ, Petersdorf RG, Wilson JD, Martin J, Fauci AS, Root RK, editors: *Harrison's principles of internal medicine*, ed 12. New York, 1991, McGraw-Hill, p. 227.

IV-27 PARANEOPLASTIC SYNDROMES

I. Endocrine
   *A. Cushing's syndrome
   *B. Hypercalcemia
   *C. Gynecomastia
   D. Hypoglycemia
   E. Hypokalemia
   F. SIADH
   G. Carcinoid syndrome
   H. Hyperthyroidism
   I. Hypocalcemia

II. Skeletal
   *A. Digital clubbing
   *B. Hypertrophic pulmonary osteoarthropathy
   C. Hyperpigmentation

III. Skin
   *A. Dermatomyositis
   *B. Acanthosis nigricans

IV. Neurology
   *A. Eaton-Lambert syndrome
   *B. Peripheral neuropathies
   *C. Subacute cerebellar degeneration
   D. Cortical degeneration
   E. Polymyositis
   F. Transverse myelitis
   G. Progressive multifocal leukoencephalopathy
   *H. Encephalomyelitis

V. Vascular
   *A. Thrombophlebitis
   *B. Marantic endocarditis
   *C. TTP

VI. Hematology
   *A. Anemia
   B. Dysproteinemia
   *C. DIC
   D. Eosinophilia
   *E. Leukocytosis
   F. Erythrocytosis
   *G. Thrombocytosis
   H. Thrombocytopenia

VII. Other
   A. Nephrotic syndrome
   B. Hypouricemia

*Associated with bronchogenic carcinoma

IV-28 CAUSES OF HYPONATREMIA IN CANCER PATIENTS

   I. Pseudohyponatremia (multiple myeloma, other paraproteinemias)
   II. Adrenal insufficiency
   III. Gastrointestinal losses with "pure water" replacement
   IV. SIADH
      A. Tumor-related (usually small cell carcinoma of the lung)
      B. Drug-related (cyclophosphamide, vinca alkaloids, narcotic analgesics, phenothiazines, barbiturates, tricyclic antidepressants)
      C. Infection-related (pulmonary and central nervous system infections)
      D. Central nervous system (space-occupying lesions, infections)

IV-29 FACTORS RELATED TO THE SURVIVAL OF PATIENTS WITH BREAST CANCER

I. Disease-free survival related to lymph node status*

Axillary nodes	% Surviving disease free	
	At 5 yr	At 10 yr
Negative	83	76
1-3 Nodes positive	50	35
≥ 4 Nodes positive	21	11

II. Recurrence risk with negative nodes†
   A. Low risk
      1. Ductal carcinoma *in situ*, pure tubular, papillary, or typical medullary types
      2. Tumor < 1 cm
      3. Diploid tumor; low S-phase fraction
   B. High risk
      1. Aneuploid tumor
      2. High S-phase fractions
      3. High cathepsin D levels
      4. Absent estrogen receptors
      5. Tumor > 3 cm

*Source: National Surgical Adjuvant Breast Project
†Modified from: McGuire R, Clark G. Prognostic factors and treatment decisions in axillary-node-negative breast cancer. *N Engl J Med* 326(26):1757, 1992.

IV-30 TNM NOMENCLATURE OF LUNG CANCERS

T x Positive sputum with normal x-ray
  1 Intraparenchymal tumor 3.0 cm or less in diameter
  2 Tumor more than 3 cm in diameter and/or invading visceral pleura or a main bronchus
  3 Any size tumor which invades chest wall, diaphragm, or mediastinal pleura
  4 Any size tumor involving heart, great vessels, esophagus, or carina, or presence of a malignant pleural effusion

N 0 No proven involvement of any lymph node
  1 Peribronchial or ipsilateral hilar node involvement
  2 Ipsilateral mediastinal or subcarinal nodes involved
  3 Contralateral mediastinal/hilar nodes, ipsilateral or contralateral scalene or supraclavicular nodes involved

M 0 No evidence of distant metastasis
  1 Distant metastasis, e.g., bone, brain, liver, etc.

IV-31 STAGES OF LUNG CANCER ACCORDING TO TNM NOMENCLATURE

Stage 0
  $T_xN_0M_0$ Occult carcinoma
*Stage I
  $T_{1-2}N_0M_0$ No lymph node involvement
*Stage II
  $T_{1-2}N_1M_0$ Intrapulmonary and/or hilar nodes involved
*Stage IIIa
  $T_3N_{0-1}M_0$ > 3 cm tumor with only peribronchial or
  $T_{1-3}N_2M_0$ ipsilateral hilar nodes involved; any size tumor not involving mediastinum with only ipsilateral subcarinal node involvement
Stage IIIb
  $T_4N_{0-2}M_0$ Any size tumor involving mediastinum or with
  $T_{1-4}N_3M_0$ contralateral node involvement
Stage IV
  $T_{x-4}N_{0-3}M_1$ Distant metastasis

*Considered potentially resectable

Adapted from: Minna J, Pass H, Glatstein E, Ihde, D. In DeVita VTJr, Hellman S, Rosenberg SA, editors: *Cancer: principles and practice of oncology*, ed 3. Philadelphia, 1989, J. B. Lippincott, p. 620.

IV-32 MOST FREQUENT TYPES OF NEOPLASMS IN MALIGNANT PLEURAL EFFUSIONS

I. Breast
II. Lung
III. Lymphoma/leukemia
IV. Ovary
V. Unknown primary
VI. GI tract
VII. Mesothelioma
VIII. Uterus
IX. Kidney
X. Sarcoma

Modified from: Papac RJ. In Becker FF, editor: *Cancer: a comprehensive treatise*, vol 5. New York, 1977, Plenum Press, p. 208.

IV-33 MOST FREQUENT MALIGNANCIES CAUSING PERITONEAL EFFUSIONS

I. Ovary
II. Stomach
III. Uterus
IV. Unknown primary
V. Breast
VI. Lymphoma
VII. Mesothelioma

Modified from: Papac RJ. In Becker FF, editor: *Cancer: a comprehensive treatise*, vol 5. New York, 1977, Plenum Press, p. 212.

IV-34 MOST FREQUENT NEOPLASMS CAUSING MALIGNANT PERICARDIAL EFFUSION

I. Leukemia, lymphoma
II. Breast
III. Lung
IV. Skin (melanoma)

Modified from: Papac RJ. In Becker FF, editor: *Cancer: a comprehensive treatise*, vol 5. New York, 1977, Plenum Press, p. 214.

IV-35 ETIOLOGIC FACTORS OF HYPERCALCEMIA OF MALIGNANCY

I. Humoral factors
   A. Parathyroid hormone (PTH)—rare
   B. PTH-like factors
   C. Transforming growth factors (TGFa, TGFb)
   D. Prostaglandins
   E. Tumor necrosis factors
   F. Platelet derived growth factor
   G. Colony-stimulating factors
   H. 1,25 dihydroxyvitamin D (with certain lymphomas)
II. Other causes
   A. Direct bone resorption by tumor—rare
   B. Increased GI absorption of calcium—rare
   C. Increased renal reabsorption of calcium

Modified from: Warrell R, Bockman R. *Cancer: principles of oncology*, ed 3, 1989, p. 1988.

IV-36 CANCERS MOST LIKE TO METASTASIZE TO BONE

I. Thyroid
II. Breast
III. Prostate
IV. Renal
V. Lung

IV-37 GENERAL RESPONSES OF VARIOUS MALIGNANCIES TO ANTINEOPLASTIC CHEMOTHERAPY

I. Chemotherapy potentially curative
   A. Acute lymphocytic leukemia of childhood
   B. Burkitt's lymphoma
   C. Gestational trophoblastic neoplasia
   D. Hodgkin's disease
   E. Non-Hodgkin's lymphomas (diffuse large cell, nodular lymphocytic, nodular mixed types)
   F. Testicular tumors
   G. Embryonal rhabdomyosarcoma of childhood
   H. Ewing's sarcoma
   I. Wilms' tumor
   J. Acute nonlymphocytic leukemia (few percent)
   K. Ovarian carcinomas (few percent)

II. Chemotherapy palliative
   A. Adrenal carcinoma
   B. Acute lymphocytic leukemia of adults
   C. Acute nonlymphocytic leukemia
   D. Breast carcinoma
   E. Chronic myelogenous leukemia
   G. Endometrial carcinoma
   H. Gastric carcinoma
   I. Glioblastoma (few percent)
   J. Islet cell tumors
   K. Medullary carcinoma of the thyroid
   L. Multiple myeloma
   M. Neuroblastoma
   N. Non-Hodgkin's lymphomas
   O. Osteosarcoma
   P. Ovarian carcinoma
   Q. Prostatic carcinoma
   R. Bronchogenic carcinomas
   S. Soft-tissue sarcomas
   T. Bladder carcinoma
   U. Head and neck carcinomas
   V. Colorectal carcinoma

III. Chemotherapy marginally or questionably beneficial
   A. Biliary tract carcinoma
   B. Brain tumors
   C. Carcinoid tumors
   D. Cervical carcinoma
   E. Hepatocellular carcinoma
   F. Malignant melanoma

IV-37 GENERAL RESPONSES OF VARIOUS MALIGNANCIES TO ANTINEOPLASTIC CHEMOTHERAPY (CONTINUED)

    G. Pancreatic carcinoma
    H. Renal cell carcinoma
    I. Thyroid carcinoma

Modified from: Moosa A, Robson M, Schimpff J. In *Comprehensive textbook of oncology, ed 2. Baltimore, 1991, Williams and Wilkins*, p. 528.

IV-38 LONG-TERM EFFECTS OF RADIATION

      I.   Salivary gland — xerostomia
     II. Esophagus — ulcer, stricture
    III. Stomach — achlorhydria, pyloric stenosis, ulceration
    IV. Small intestine — ulcer, perforation, stricture, malabsorption
     V. Colon — ulcer, perforation, stricture, fistula formation
    VI. Kidney — nephritis
   VII. Bladder — ulceration, contracture, dysuria, frequency
  VIII. Lung — pneumonitis, fibrosis
    IX. Heart — pericarditis, pancarditis
     X. Bone — arrested growth - children
    XI. CNS — atrophy
   XII. Spinal cord — transverse myelitis

Modified from: Becker FF, editor: *Cancer: a comprehensive treatise*, vol 5. New York, 1977, Plenum Press, p. 8.

IV-39 CLINICAL FEATURES OF GRAFT-VERSUS-HOST DISEASE

I. Suggested clinical staging

Stage	Skin	Liver	Intestinal tract
+	Maculopapular rash < 25% body surface	Serum bilirubin 2-3 mg/dl	> 500 ml stool volume/day
++	Maculopapular rash 25% to 50% body surface	Serum bilirubin 3-6 mg/dl	> 1000 ml stool volume/day
+++	Generalized erythroderma	Serum bilirubin 6-15 mg/dl	> 1500 ml stool volume/day
++++	Generalized erythroderma; bullous formation; desquamation	Serum bilirubin > 15 mg/dl	Severe abdominal pain; ileus

II. Suggested overall clinical grading

Grade	Skin	Liver	GI tract	Survival
I	+ — + +	0	0	> 50%
II	+ — + + +	+	+	
III	+ + — + + +	+ + — + + +	+ + — + + +	15%
IV	+ + — + + + +	+ + — + + + +	+ + — + + + +	15%

Reference: Thomas ED. *New Engl J Med* 292:895, 1975.

IV-40 SUPERIOR VENA CAVA SYNDROME

    I. Neoplasm
      A. 90% lung carcinoma
      B. 10% lymphoma
    II. Mediastinitis
      A. Fibrosing (TB, histoplasmosis, syphilis, pyogenic)
      B. Idiopathic
      C. Methysergide
   III. Aortic aneurysm
   IV. Thrombophlebitis
    V. Constrictive pericarditis
   VI. Retrosternal thyroid
  VII. Central venous catheters

IV-41 CAUDA EQUINA SYNDROME

    I. Perineal, buttock, leg pain
    II. Sphincteric incontinence
   III. Loss of sensation in perineum, posterior thigh, lateral feet
   IV. ↓ DTR's
    V. Foot drop
   VI. Impotence

IV-42 SIGNS AND SYMPTOMS OF METASTATIC EPIDURAL COMPRESSION

    I. Pain — 96%
    II. Weakness — 76%
   III. Autonomic dysfunction — 57%
   IV. Sensory disturbances — 51%
    V. Ataxia - 3%
   VI. Flexor spasms — 2%

Adapted from: Byrne T. Spinal cord compression from epidural metastases. *N Engl J Med* 327(6):614, Aug. 27, 1992.

IV-43 COTSWOLD STAGING CLASSIFICATION OF HODGKIN'S DISEASE

Stage I   Single lymph node region or lymphoid structure involved
Stage II   Two or more lymph node regions on the same side of the diaphragm involved (number of anatomical sites indicated by a subscript)
Stage III   Lymph node regions on both sides of the diaphragm involved
   III_1 With or without splenic, hilar, celiac, or portal node involvement
   III_2 Para-aortic, iliac, and mesenteric nodes involved
Stage IV   One or more extranodal sites involved (in addition to a site for which the designation "E" has been used)

Designations:
   A   No symptoms
   B   Fever (> 38°C), night sweats, unexplained weight loss > 10% within last 6 months
   X   Bulky disease (widening of mediastinum by more than one-third or a nodal mass greater than 10 cm)
   E   Involvement of a single extranodal site that is contiguous or proximal to the known nodal site.

Modified from: Urbu W, Longo D. Medical progress: Hodgkin's disease, *N Engl J Med* 326(10):679, March 5, 1992.

IV-44 WORKING FORMULATION OF NON-HODGKIN'S LYMPHOMAS

Rappeport
terminology

1. Malignant lymphoma
   Small lymphocytic   DWDL
      Consistent with chronic
      lymphocytic leukemia
2. Malignant lymphoma, follicular
   Predominantly small cleaved cell   NPDL
      Diffuse areas
      Sclerosis
3. Malignant lymphoma, follicular
   Mixed, small cleaved, and large cell   NML
      Diffuse areas
      Sclerosis

Intermediate grade

4. Malignant lymphoma, follicular
   Predominantly large cell   NHL
      Diffuse areas
      Sclerosis
5. Malignant lymphoma, diffuse
   Small cleaved cell   DPDL
      Sclerosis
6. Malignant lymphoma, diffuse
   Mixed, small, and large cell   DML
      Sclerosis
      Epithelioid-cell component
7. Malignant lymphoma, diffuse
   Large cell   DHL
   Cleaved cell
      Noncleaved cell
      Sclerosis

High grade

8. Malignant lymphoma
   Large cell, immunoblastic   DHL
      Plasmacytoid
      Clear cell
      Polymorphous
      Epithelioid-cell component
9. Malignant lymphoma
   Lymphoblastic   Lymphoblastic
      Convoluted cell
      Nonconvoluted cell

IV-44 WORKING FORMUATION OF NON-HODGKIN'S LYMPHOMAS (CONTINUED)

	Rappeport terminology
10. Malignant lymphoma	
Small noncleaved cell	DUL
Burkitt's lymphoma	
Follicular areas	
Miscellaneous	
Composite	
Histiocytic	
Extramedullary plasmacytoma	
Unclassifiable	
Other	

DWDL = diffuse, well-differentiated, lymphocytic
NPDL = nodular, poorly-differentiated, lymphocytic
NML = nodular, mixed lymphocytic-histiocytic
NHL = nodular histiocytic
DPDL = diffuse, poorly-differentiated, lymphocytic
DML = diffuse, mixed lymphocytic-histiocytic
DHL = diffuse histiocytic
DUL = undifferentiated

Source: Moose A, Robson M, Schimpff J. *Comprehensive textbook of oncology.* Baltimore, 1986, Williams & Wilkins, p. 577.

IV-45 PERFORMANCE STATUS CRITERIA (KARNOFSKY SCALE)

Able to carry on normal activity; no special care needed	100	Normal; no complaints; no evidence of disease
	90	Able to carry on normal activity; minor signs or symptoms of disease
	80	Normal activity with some effort; some signs or symptoms of disease
Unable to work; able to live at home and care for most personal needs; a varying amount of assistance is needed	70	Cares for self; unable to carry on normal activity or to do active work
	60	Requires occasional care for most needs
	50	Requires considerable assistance and frequent medical care
Unable to care for self; requires equivalent of institutional or hospital care; disease may be progressing rapidly	40	Disabled; requires special care and assistance
	30	Severely disabled; hospitalization is indicated although death not imminent
	20	Very sick; hospitalization; active supportive treatment is necessary
	10	Moribund, fatal processes progressing rapidly
	0	Dead

Source: Moose A, Robson M, Schimpff J. *Comprehensive textbook of oncology.* Baltimore, 1986, Williams & Wilkins, p. 67.

IV-46 MULTIPLE ENDOCRINE NEOPLASIA SYNDROME

I. Multiple endocrine neoplasia type I (MEN I)
   A. Parathyroid neoplasia or hyperplasia (hyperparathyroidism)
   B. Pancreatic islet cell neoplasms (insulin, gastrin, VIP)
   C. Pituitary neoplasms (acromegaly, nonfunctioning tumors)
   D. Adrenal cortical neoplasms or hyperplasia (Cushing's syndrome)
   E. Thyroid involvement (hyperthyroidism; nonfunctional adenomas)
   F. About 2/3 of patients have adenomas of two or more systems and 1/5 develop adenoma in three or more systems
II. Multiple endocrine neoplasia type II (MEN II A)
   A. Pheochromocytoma
   B. Medullary carcinoma of the thyroid
   C. Parathyroid neoplasm or hyperplasia
III. Multiple endocrine neoplasia type III (MEN II B)
   A. Medullary carcinoma of the thyroid
   B. Pheochromocytoma
   C. Dysmorphic features (ganglioneuroma or neuromas of conjunctiva, buccal mucosa, tongue, larynx, gastrointestinal tract)

IV-47 RISK FACTORS PREDISPOSING TO THROMBOSIS

I. Genetic predisposition
  A. Abnormal fibrin formation
    1. Antithrombin III deficiency
    2. Heparin cofactor II deficiency
    3. Protein C deficiency
    4. Protein S deficiency
    5. Fibrinogen deficiency
  B. Abnormal fibrinolysis
    1. Plasminogen deficiency
    2. α_2-antiplasmin deficiency
    3. Plasminogen activator deficiency
    4. Plasminogen activator inhibitor present
  C. Disorder of vascular injury
    1. Homocystinemia
II. Venous thrombosis
  A. Increased venous stasis: immobilization, pregnancy, CHF, varicosities, obesity
  B. Coagulation activation: trauma, surgery, malignancies, lupus inhibitor, myocardial infarction, Factor IX concentrates
III. Arterial thrombosis
  A. Abnormal vascular surface: atherosclerosis, hyperlipidemia, diabetes, hypertension, cigarette smoking, estrogen therapy
  B. Vascular occlusion: hyperviscosity, sickle cell disease, polycythemia, plasma cell dyscrasias (especially macroglobulinemia)
  C. Increased platelet reactivity: thrombocytosis

Adapted from: Harker, L. In Williams WJ, Beutler E, Erslev AJ, Lichtman MA, editors: *Hematology*, ed 4. New York, 1990, McGraw-Hill, pp. 1565-1567.

CHAPTER V
INFECTIOUS DISEASE

V-1 DISEASE STATES CAUSING FEVER OF UNKNOWN ORIGIN (FUO)*

I. Infection
  A. Generalized
    1. Tuberculosis
    2. Histoplasmosis
    3. Typhoid fever
    4. CMV
    5. EB virus
    6. Miscellaneous: syphilis, brucellosis, toxoplasmosis, malaria
    7. HIV
  B. Localized
    1. Infective endocarditis
    2. Empyema
    3. Intraabdominal infection
       a. Peritonitis
       b. Cholangitis
       c. Abscess
    4. Urinary tract
       a. Pyelonephritis
       b. Perinephric abscess
       c. Prostatitis
    5. Decubitus ulcer
    6. Osteomyelitis
    7. Thrombophlebitis
II. Neoplasm
  A. Hematological
    1. Lymphoma
    2. Hodgkin's disease
    3. Acute leukemia
  B. Tumors predisposed to cause fever
    1. Hepatoma
    2. Hypernephroma
    3. Atrial myxoma
III. Connective tissue disease
  A. RA, SLE
  B. Vasculitis
IV. Miscellaneous
  A. Drug induced
  B. Immune complex: SLE, RA
  C. Vasculitis
  D. Alcoholic liver disease
  E. Granulomatous hepatitis
  F. Inflammatory bowel disease, Whipple's disease

V-1 DISEASE STATES CAUSING FEVER OF UNKNOWN ORIGIN (FUO)*(CONTINUED)

  G. Recurrent pulmonary emboli
  H. Factitious fever
  I. Undiagnosed

*Diagnostic criteria for FUO
  1. Illness of more than three weeks duration
  2. Fever, intermittent or continuous
  3. Documentation of fever > 38.3°C
  4. No obvious diagnosis after initial complete examination
Approximate current breakdown:
  1. Neoplasms — 7.0%
  2. Infections — 22.7%
  3. Multisystem diseases — 21.5%
  4. Miscellaneous — 14.5%
  5. No diagnosis — 25.6%

Modified from: Knockaert DC, et al. *Arch Intern Med* 1992; 152:51-55.

V-2 CLASSIFICATION OF TUBERCULOSIS

  I. Tuberculosis exposure, no evidence of infection
  II. Tuberculosis infection, no evidence of disease
   A. Chemotherapy status
  III. Tuberculosis
   A. Location
   B. Bacteriological status
   C. Chemotherapy status

V-3 CLINICAL FEATURES OF GENITOURINARY TUBERCULOSIS

Sterile pyuria	50%
Painless hematuria	40%
Fever	10%
Perinephric abscess	10%
+ sputum culture	20% to 40%
+ urine culture	80%

Reference: Smith AM, Lattimer JK. Genitourinary tract involvement in children with tuberculosis. *NY State J Med* 73:235, 1973.

V-4 CRITERIA FOR THE DIAGNOSIS OF NONTUBERCULOSIS MYCOBACTERIAL DISEASE IN NONIMMUNOCOMPROMISED HOSTS

I. The patient should have clinical evidence of disease compatible with the diagnosis.
II. Isolation of the organism in colony counts of more than 100 on four or more occasions (with the exception of M. kansasii)
III. Isolation of the organism from ordinarily sterile sources
IV. Culture of the organism from a biopsy specimen
V. Check HIV status

Adapted from: Davidson PT. The management of disease with atypical mycobacteria. *Clin Notes Respir*, Summer 1979, pp. 3-13.
Adapted from: Tellis CJ, et al. *Med Clin North Am* 64(3):437, May 1980.

V-5 IMMUNOCOMPROMISED HOSTS

I. Hematologic malignancy (leukemia, lymphoma, multiple myeloma)
II. Solid tumors
III. Transplant recipients (renal, heart, heart-lung, liver, bone marrow)
IV. Corticosteroid therapy
V. Immunosuppressive agents
VI. Alcoholics
VII. Cirrhosis
VIII. Chronic renal failure
IX. Diabetes mellitus
X. Intravenous drug abusers
XI. Elderly
XII. AIDS
XIII. Post-splenectomy
XIV. Burns
XV. Malnutrition
XVI. Sickle cell anemia
XVII. Infants

V-6 PULMONARY INFECTIONS IN IMMUNOCOMPROMISED PATIENTS

I. Bacteria
   A. Pseudomonas
   B. Klebsiella
   C. Serratia
   D. Nocardia
   E. Tuberculosis
   F. Listeria
II. Fungal
   A. Aspergillus
   B. Candida
   C. Coccidioidomycosis
   D. Cryptococcosis
   E. Phycomycetes
   F. Histoplasmosis
III. Viral
   A. CMV
   B. Herpes simplex
   C. Varicella-zoster
   D. Measles
   E. Adenovirus
   F. Legionella pneumophilia
IV. Protozoa
   A. Pneumocystis
   B. Toxoplasma

Adapted from: Matthay RA, Green WH. Pulmonary infections in the immunocompromised patient. *Med Clin North Am* 64:534, 1980.

V-7 CLINICAL PULMONARY SYNDROMES OF HISTOPLASMOSIS

I. Primary pulmonary histoplasmosis
II. Histoplasmoma
III. Fibrosing mediastinitis
IV. Disseminated histoplasmosis
V. Chronic cavitary fibronodular pulmonary histoplasmosis

V-8 EXTRAPULMONARY MANIFESTATIONS OF MYCOPLASMA PNEUMONIAE

I. Hematological
   A. Autoimmune hemolytic anemia
   B. Thrombocytopenia
   C. DIC
   D. Splenomegaly
II. Gastrointestinal
   A. Gastroenteritis
   B. Anicteric hepatitis
   C. Pancreatitis
III. Musculoskeletal
   A. Arthralgias
   B. Myalgias
   C. Polyarthritis
IV. Cardiac
   A. Pericarditis
   B. Myocarditis
   C. Conduction defects
   D. Pericardial effusion
V. Neurological
   A. Meningitis
   B. Meningoencephalitis
   C. Transverse myelitis
   D. Peripheral and cranial neuropathies
   E. Cerebellar ataxia
VI. Dermatological
   A. Erythema nodosum
   B. Erythema multiforme
   C. Stevens-Johnson
VII. Renal
   A. Interstitial nephritis
   B. Glomerulonephritis

Adapted from: Murray HW, Tuazon C. Atypical pneumonias. *Med Clin North Am* 564:512, 1980.

V-9 EXTRAPULMONARY MANIFESTATIONS OF PSITTACOSIS

I. Cardiac
   A. Myocarditis
   B. Pericarditis
   C. Endocarditis
II. Neurological
   A. Meningitis
   B. Encephalitis
   C. Seizure
III. Hematological
   A. Anemia, non-hemolytic
   B. Hemolytic anemia
   C. DIC
   D. Splenomegaly
IV. Gastrointestinal
   A. Hepatitis
   B. Pancreatitis
V. Renal
   A. Nephritis
   B. Acute renal failure
   C. Proteinuria

Adapted from: Murray HW, Tuazon C. Atypical pneumonias. *Med Clin North Am* 64:517, 1980.

V-10 EXTRAPULMONARY MANIFESTATIONS OF Q FEVER

I. Gastrointestinal
   A. Hepatitis
II. Cardiovascular
   A. Pericarditis
   B. Myocarditis
   C. Endocarditis
   D. Pericardial effusion
   E. Thrombophlebitis
   F. Arteritis
III. Ocular
   A. Uveitis
   B. Iritis
   C. Optic neuritis
IV. Neurological
   A. Meningitis
   B. Peripheral neuropathy

Adapted from: Murray HW, Tuazon C. Atypical pneumonias. *Med Clin North Am* 64:521, 1980.

V-11 FEATURES OF LEGIONELLA INFECTION

I. Pneumonia-bronchopneumonia with pleuritis, pleural effusion rare
   A. Fever — often high with rigors and chills > 90%
   B. Nonproductive cough 90%
   C. Nausea/emesis
   D. Diarrhea with abdominal pain 30% to 50%
   E. Mental status changes 30%
      1. Lethargy
      2. Confusion
      3. Emotional lability
      4. Slurred speech
      5. Hallucination
      6. Seizures
      7. Coma
      8. Cerebellar dysfunction
      9. Peripheral neuropathy
      10. Motor weakness
   F. Myalgias
   G. Rash — macular
   H. Ocular-Roth and cotton wool exudates
   I. Lab: ↑WBC, L shift
           ↓Na, ↓PO_4
           ↑AST, alk phos, LDH
II. Wound infection
III. Dialysis shunt infection
IV. Sinusitis
V. Pericarditis

Poor prognosticators: RR > 30, HR > 110, WBC > 14,000, Bands > 10%, renal failure, bilateral pulmonary involvement, hypoxemia

References: Meyer RD. *Rev. Infect. Dis.* 5:258, 1983. Swartz MN. *Ann Intern Med* 90:492, 1979.

V-12 CLINICAL AND LABORATORY FEATURES OF CYTOMEGALOVIRUS MONONUCLEOSIS* (NON-IMMUNE COMPROMISED HOST)

Clinical	Estimated percent positive
I. Clinical	
A. Prolonged fever (>4 weeks)	20*
B. Hepatomegaly	30-50
C. Splenomegaly	30-50
D. Pharyngitis	5
E. Lymphadenopathy	10
II. Laboratory	
A. Lymphocytosis (>50% of cells)	98
B. Atypical lymphocytes (>20% of lymphocytes)	90
C. Rheumatoid factor, cryoglobulin	30
D. Cold agglutinin (anti-I or anti-i)	25
E. Antinuclear factor	20
F. Coombs' test	10
G. Fourfold CMV CF antibody change	85
H. Virus isolation:	
1. Urine	50-60
2. Saliva	70-80
I. Simultaneous infection with	
1. Epstein-Barr virus	5

*Fever of 2 weeks duration was the criterion for inclusion.

Reference: Betts RF. In Stollerman GH, editor: *Advances in internal medicine*, vol 26. Chicago, 1980, Year Book Medical Publishers, Chicago, p. 455.

V-13 FACTORS ASSOCIATED WITH MORTALITY IN BRAIN ABSCESS

    I. Coma on admission
   II. Multiple brain abscesses
  III. Rupture of abscess in ventricle
  IV. Inaccurate or missed diagnosis
   V. Positive spinal fluid cultures
  VI. Brain abscess secondary to remote focus of infection
 VII. Absence of focal signs
VIII. Seizures
  IX. Symptoms of meningitis early in the illness

Reference: Karandanis D, Shulman JA. Factors associated with mortality in brain abscess. *Arch Intern Med* 135:1145, 1975.

V-14 RISK FACTORS AFFECTING OUTCOME OF BACTEREMIA

   I. Male gender with age > 75 years.
  II. Azotemia (creatinine > 2.0 mg/dl)
 III. Pseudomonas species
 IV. *Streptococcus pneumoniae*
  V. Absence of fever (< 38°)
 VI. Coagulopathy
 VII. Interstitial pattern on chest x-ray involving more than half of both lung fields
VIII. Delayed, inappropriate, or inadequate levels of antibiotics
 IX. Underlying immunosuppression
    A. Antecedent antimetabolites
    B. Antecedent corticosteroids
    C. Asplenia
    D. Diabetes mellitus
    E. Human immunodeficiency virus
  X. Lactic acidosis

Modified from: Kreger BE, et al. *Am J Med* 68:344, 1980 and Aube H, et al. *Am J Med* 93:283, 1992.

V-15 MAJOR TYPES OF OSTEOMYELITIS*

Feature	Hematogenous	Secondary to Contiguous Focus of Infection	Due to Vascular Insufficiency
I. Age distribution (yr)	Peaks at 1-20 and ≥50	≥50	≥50
II. Bones involved	Long bones Vertebrae	Femur, tibia, skull, mandible	Feet
III. Precipitating factors	Trauma (?) Bacteremia	Surgery Soft-tissue infections Often mixed infection	Diabetes mellitus Peripheral vascular disease Usually mixed infections
IV. Bacteriology	Usually only one organism S. aureus Gram-negative organisms	S. aureus Gram-negative organisms Anaerobic organisms	S. aureus or epidermidis Streptococci Gram-negative organisms Anaerobic organisms
V. Episode Major clinical findings	Initial Fever Local tenderness Local swelling Limitation of motion	Initial Fever Erythema Swelling Heat	Initial and Recurrent Pain Swelling Erythema Drainage Ulceration
	Recurrent Drainage	Recurrent Drainage Sinus	

V-15 MAJOR TYPES OF OSTEOMYELITIS* (CONTINUED)
Bacteriology of Prosthetic Joint Infection†

Pathogens	Frequency (%)
Staphylococci	53
S. epidermidis	28
S. aureus	25
Streptococci	20
β-Hemolytic streptococci	12
Viridans streptococci	8
Gram-negative aerobic bacilli	20
Anaerobes	7

*From: Norden CW. In Mandell GL, Douglas RG, Bennett JE, editors: *Principles and Practice of Infectious Disease*, ed 3. New York, 1990, Churchill-Livingstone, p. 922-30.

†From: Brause BD. In Mandell GL, Douglas RG, Bennett JE, editors: *Principles and practice of infectious disease*, ed 3. New York, 1990, Churchill-Livingstone, p. 919.

184

V-16 SPECTRUM OF GONOCOCCAL INFECTIONS

I. Urethritis
II. Cervicitis
III. Prostatitis
IV. Epididymitis
V. Pelvic inflammatory disease
VI. Salpingitis
VII. Proctitis
VIII. Conjunctivitis
IX. Pharyngitis
X. Dermatitis
XI. Arthritis
XII. Perihepatitis
XIII. Peritonitis
XIV. Pericarditis
XV. Myocarditis
XVI. Endocarditis
XVII. Hepatitis
XVIII. Meningitis

V-17 CLINICAL FEATURES OF FOOD POISONING SECONDARY TO BOTULISM

    I. Visual disturbances (mydriasis, ophthalmoplegia, diplopia)
    II. Speech disturbances (dysphonia, dysarthria)
    III. Dysphagia
    IV. Descending motor paralysis, bilaterally symmetrical
    V. Clear sensorium
    VI. Fever is unusual
    VII. Diarrhea is rare, constipation is the rule

Reference: Thadepalli H. In Thadepalli MD, editor: *Infectious diseases. Focus on clinical diagnosis*, Garden City, New York, 1980, Medical Examination Publishing.

V-18 ANTIBIOTIC-ASSOCIATED PSEUDOMEMBRANOUS COLITIS

I. Antibiotics implicated
   *Lincomycin
   *Amoxicillin
   Erythromycin
   Neomycin
   *Clindamycin
   *Cephalosporins
   Oral penicillin
   Vancomycin
   *Ampicillin
   Tetracycline
   Gentamicin
   Sulfamethoxazol/etrimethorprim
   Quinolones

II. Clinical features
   A. Diarrhea (rarely bloody)
   B. Crampy abdominal pain and tenderness to palpation
   C. Fever
   D. Toxic megacolon (rare)
   E. Leukocytosis

III. Diagnosis
   A. Pseudomembranous lesion (plaques) visualized at sigmoidoscopy (75% to 80% of cases)
   B. Demonstration of *C. difficile* toxin

IV. Treatment
   A. Discontinue antibiotics
   B. Metronidazole or vancomycin — 10% to 15% of patients will relapse after treatment
   C. Bile salt sequestering agents (cholestyramine)

*Especially important

V-19 TOXIC SHOCK SYNDROME

I. Etiology and epidemiology
A. Approximately 50% of cases occur in women < 30 years of age
B. 50% of cases not associated with menstruation (1/3 are men)
1. Drug abusers
2. Homosexuals
3. Staphylococcal/streptococcal sepsis
4. Surgical wound infections
5. Nonsurgical traumatic wounds
6. Parturition
7. Staphylococcal/streptococcal pneumonia
C. Strong correlation between toxic shock syndrome and recovery of *S. aureus* from vaginal cultures
D. Toxins elaborated by *S. aureus* (TSST-1) and group A streptococcus exotoxin A are responsible for the clinical manifestations

II. Clinical features
A. Multisystem disease
1. Rash — macular, erythematous, often desquamative
2. Fever
3. Hypotension
4. Desquamation — 1 to 2 weeks after illness onset, particularly of palms and soles
5. Volume depletion
6. Renal insufficiency
7. Liver test abnormalities
8. Nausea, vomiting, diarrhea
9. Thrombocytopenia, subclinical DIC
10. Disorientation with/without focal neurological signs
11. Mucous membranes — hyperemia
B. Diagnosis
1. No. 1-4 and any 3 of items No. 5-11 or
No. 1-3 and any 5 of items No. 5-11

III. Differential diagnosis
A. Meningococcemia
B. Rocky Mountain spotted fever
C. Leptospirosis
D. Drug eruption
E. Rubella

Adapted from: Bone RC, Barkoviak J. *J Crit Illness* 1992: 7(7):1032-1044.

V-20 ANAEROBIC INFECTIONS

I. Host factors that may predispose to development of anaerobic infection
   A. Disruption of normal cutaneous or mucosal barriers
   B. Tissue injury (accidental trauma, surgery, or invasive diagnostic procedure)
   C. Impaired blood supply (including microvascular disease)
   D. Tissue necrosis
   E. Obstruction of hollow viscus (tracheobronchial tree, biliary tract, gastrointestinal tract, fallopian tube)
   F. Presence of foreign body
   G. Underlying malignancy

II. Clinical clues to anaerobic infections
   A. Foul order of lesion or discharge
   B. Location of infection in proximity to mucosal surface
   C. Tissue necrosis; abscess formation
   D. Infection secondary to human or animal bite
   E. Gas in tissues or discharges
   F. Classical clinical picture such as gas gangrene
   G. Previous therapy with aminoglycoside antibiotics (e.g., neomycin, gentamicin, and amikacin)
   H. Black discoloration or red fluorescence under UV light of blood containing exudates (pigmented *Bacteroides* infection)
   I. Septic thrombophlebitis
   J. Presence of "sulfur granules" in discharges (actinomycosis)
   K. Unique morphology on Gram stain of exudate (pleomorphic or otherwise distinctive)
   L. Failure of culture to grow aerobically, organisms seen on Gram stain of original exudate

III. Source of anaerobic bacteremia by portal of entry (n = 40)
   A. Gastrointestinal tract — 60%
   B. Skin — 15%
   C. Genitourinary tract — 8%
   D. Oral — 2%
   E. Uncertain —13%

Reference: Finegold SM, George WL, Mulligan ME. Anaerobic infections. In Cotsonas NJ, editor: *Disease-a-month*, ed 31. Chicago, 1985, Year Book Medical Publishers,10:21,26.
Modified from: Lombardi DP, Engleberg NC. *Am J Med* 1992;92:53-60.

V-21 LISTERIA MONOCYTOGENES INFECTIONS

I. Presentations
   A. Meningoencephalitis
   B. Septicemia
   C. Endocarditis
   D. Endophthalmitis
   E. Peritonitis
   F. Pleurisy
   G. Osteomyelitis
   H. Lymphadenitis
   I. Conjunctivitis
   J. Cholecystitis
   K. Visceral abscesses
   L. Amnionitis
II. Predisposing factors
   A. Malignancy
   B. Immunosuppression
   C. Alcoholism
   D. Diabetes
   E. Chronic hepatic disease
   F. Pregnancy
   G. AIDS

Adapted from: Nieman RE, Lorber B. Listeriosis in adults: a changing pattern. Report of eight cases and review of the literature, 1968-1978. *Rev. Infect. Dis.* 2:207, 1980.

References: *MMWR* 31:207, 513.

V-22 EFFECTIVE DRUG REGIMENS FOR THE TREATMENT OF TUBERCULOSIS*

Regimen (adult drug dose)	Comment
Isoniazid (300 mg) and rifampin (600 mg) daily for 9-12 months	The usual regimen for initial treatment of all patients unless drug resistance is suspected, in which case ethambutol 15 mg/kg should be added.
Isoniazid (300 mg) and ethambutol (15 mg/kg) daily for 12-18 months	The least toxic effective regimen. Suitable for patients with minimal disease. The regimen of choice in pregnant women.
Isoniazid (300 mg) and thioacetazone (150 mg) daily for 12-18 months	The least expensive effective regimen. Streptomycin (0.75-1 g) may be added daily for the first 8 weeks to to increase effectiveness, but this doubles both cost and toxicity.
Isoniazid (300 mg), rifampin (600 mg), pyrazinamide (2 g), and streptomycin (1 g) or ethambutol (15 mg/kg) daily for 2 months followed by one of the following: a. Isoniazid (300 gm) and rifampin (600 gm) daily for 4 months	Initial intensive phase for short course regimens. Short course regimens have only been demonstrated to be effective under conditions of close patient supervision.

V-22 EFFECTIVE DRUG REGIMENS FOR THE TREATMENT OF TUBERCULOSIS* (CONTINUED)

Regimen (adult drug dose)	Comment
b. Isoniazid (300 mg) and Thioacetazone (150 mg) daily for 6 months	Inexpensive.
c. Isoniazid (300 mg), rifampin (600 mg), and streptomycin (1 g) twice weekly for 6 months	Suitable for fully supervised therapy.
Isoniazid (300 mg), rifampin (600 mg) daily for 1 month followed by isoniazid (900 mg) and rifampin (600 mg) twice weekly for 8 months	Effectiveness demonstrated in ambulatory treatment programs in Arkansas. Has not been compared with other regimens in clinical trials.

*With recent outbreaks of multidrug resistant tuberculosis, some authors suggest a minimum initial treatment of 4 drugs (isoniazid, rifampin, pyrazinamide and ethambutol or streptomycin). If multidrug resistant organism is suspected, additional drugs should be given based on suspected susceptibilities.
Reference: Dooley SW, et al. Ann Intern Med 117(3):257, 1992.

Source: Daniel TM. Tuberculosis. In Braunwald E, Isselbacher KJ, Petersdorf RG, Wilson JD, Martin J, Fauci AS, Root RK, editors: Harrison's principles of internal medicine, ed 12. New York, 1991, McGraw-Hill, p. 643.

V-23 MANIFESTATIONS OF LYME DISEASE BY STAGE*

	Localized (Stage I)	Early infection disseminated (Stage II)	Late infection persistent (Stage III)
I. Skin	Erythema migrans	Secondary annular lesions, malar rash, diffuse erythema or urticaria, evanescent lesions, lymphocytoma	Acrodermatitis chronica atrophicans, localized scleroderma-like lesions
II. Musculoskeletal system		Migratory pain in joints, tendons, bursae, muscle, bone; brief arthritis attacks; myositis‡, osteomyelitis‡, panniculitis‡	Prolonged arthritis attacks, chronic arthritis, peripheral enthesopathy, periostitis or joint subluxations below lesions of acrodermatitis
III. Neurologic system		Meningitis, cranial neuritis, Bell's palsy, motor or sensory radiculoneuritis, subtle encephalitis, mononeuritis multiplex, myelitis‡, chorea‡, cerebellar ataxia‡	Chronic encephalomyelitis, spastic parapareses, ataxic gait, subtle mental disorders, chronic axonal polyradiculopathy, dementia‡
IV. Lymphatic system	Regional lymph-adenopathy	Regional or generalized lymphadenopathy, splenomegaly	
V. Heart		Atrioventricular nodal block, myopericarditis, pancarditis	

V-23 MANIFESTATIONS OF LYME DISEASE BY STAGE* (CONTINUED)

	Localized (Stage I)	Early infection disseminated (Stage II)	Late infection persistent (Stage III)
VI. Eyes		Conjunctivitis, iritis‡, choroiditis‡, retinal hemorrhage or detachment‡, panophthalmitis‡	Keratitis
VII. Liver		Mild or recurrent hepatitis	
VIII. Respiratory system		Nonexudative sore throat, nonproductive cough, adult respiratory distress syndrome‡	
IX. Kidney		Microscopic hematuria or proteinuria	
X. Genitourinary system		Orchitis‡	
XI. Constitutional minor symptoms		Severe malaise and fatigue	Fatigue

*The classification by stages provides a guideline for the expected timing of the illness's manifestations, but this may vary from case to case.
†Systems are listed from the most to the least commonly affected.
‡The inclusion of this manifestation is based on one or a few cases.

Reference: Steere AC. *Engl J Med* 321(9)586-596, 1989.

V-24 CHRONIC FATIGUE SYNDROME: DIAGNOSTIC CRITERIA*

I. Major criteria

A. New onset of persistent or relapsing, debilitating fatigue in a person without a previous history of such symptoms that does not resolve with bedrest and that is severe enough to reduce or impair average daily activity to less than 50% of the patient's premorbid activity level for at least 6 months.

B. Fatigue that is not explained by the presence of other evident medical or psychiatric illness (see below).

	Illness category	Exclusions	Inclusions*	Recommended tests†
1.	Chronic medical conditions	Major conditions to be considered in differential diagnosis include malignancy, autoimmune disease, inflammatory disease, endocrine disease, neurologic disease, and chronic organic disease		Standard: Urinalysis, complete blood count with differential serum electrolytes, blood urea nitrogen, glucose, creatinine, calcium, thyroid function tests, erythrocyte sedimentation rate, and antinuclear antibodies
			Fibromyalgia‡	Tender-point examination‡ Optional or as clinically indicated: Serum cortisol, rheumatoid factor and immunoglobulin levels
2.	Postinfectious disease	Chronic active hepatitis B or C; Lyme borreliosis, inadequately treated; HIV infection; tuberculosis	Infectious mononucleosis; adequately treated infection that is not typically associated with chronicity; toxoplasmosis, brucellosis, Lyme borreliosis§	Tuberculin skin test, Lyme serology in endemic area, HIV serology when indicated

V-24 CHRONIC FATIGUE SYNDROME: DIAGNOSTIC CRITERIA* (CONTINUED)

Illness category	Exclusions	Inclusions*	Recommended tests†
3. Psychiatric and behavioral disorders	Psychoses: psychotic depression, bipolar disorder, schizophrenia Substance abuse	Nonpsychotic depression: concurrent, 1 month postonset or 6 months or more before onset: recurrent or nonrecurrent, somatoform disorders, anxiety disorders: generalized or panic disorder	Screen: General Health Questionnaire or combination of self-report instruments¶ For patients with positive screening results: Structured interview: Diagnostic Interview Schedule version III A or Structured Clinical Interview for the *Diagnostic and Statistical Manual of Mental Disorders Third Edition Revised* (DSM-III-R)

*Stratified by individual category in analysis.
†Tests are to be used in conjunction with complete detailed medical history and comprehensive physical examination
‡See Wolfe, et al. Criteria for fibromyalgia [Abstract]. *Arthritis Rheum* 1989;32(Suppl):S47.
§Recognized recrudescence and chronicity of active Borrelia infection was considered an exception.
¶Zung Self-rating Anxiety Scale, Symptom Checklist-90, Beck Depression Inventory.

V-24 CHRONIC FATIGUE SYNDROME: DIAGNOSTIC CRITERIA* (CONTINUED)

II. The minor criteria are:

At least six symptoms plus at least two signs, or at least eight symptoms from the list below

A. Symptoms:
1. Mild fever or chills
2. Sore throat
3. Painful adenopathy (posterior or anterior, cervical or axillary)
4. Generalized muscle weakness
5. Myalgias
6. Prolonged generalized fatigue after previously tolerated levels of physical activity.
7. Generalized headaches
8. Migratory arthralgia without swelling or redness
9. Neuropsychologic complaints
10. Sleep disturbance
11. Main symptom complex developing over a few hours to a few days

B. Physical signs:
1. Low-grade fever
2. Nonexudative pharyngitis
3. Palpable or tender anterior or posterior, cervical or axillary lymph nodes

*Definite diagnosis requires fulfilling of major criteria 1 and 2 *and* the following minor criteria: $\geq$ 6/11 symptoms and $\geq$ 2/3 physical signs; or $\geq$ 8/11 symptoms criteria.

Adapted from: Schluederberg A, et al. *Ann Intern Med* 117(4):325-331, 1992.

CHAPTER VI
NEPHROLOGY

VI-1 DIFFERENTIAL DIAGNOSIS OF METABOLIC ALKALOSIS

I. Sodium chloride-responsive (U_{Cl} < 10 mmoles per liter)
   A. Gastrointestinal disorders:
      1. Vomiting
      2. Gastric drainage
      3. Villous adenoma of the colon
   B. Diuretic therapy
   C. Rapid correction of chronic hypercapnia
   D. Cystic fibrosis
II. Sodium chloride-resistant (U_{Cl} > 20 mmoles per liter)
   A. Excess mineralocorticoid activity
      1. Hyperaldosteronism
      2. Cushing's syndrome
      3. Bartter's syndrome
      4. Excess licorice intake
   B. Profound potassium depletion
III. Unclassified
   A. Alkali administration
   B. Milk-alkali syndrome
   C. Nonparathyroid hypercalcemia
   D. Massive transfusion
   E. Glucose ingestion after starvation
   F. Large doses of carbenicillin or penicillin
   G. Recovery from organic acidosis
   H. Antacids and exchange resins in renal failure

Modified from: Kaehny WB, Shapiro JI. In Schrier RW, editor: *Renal and electrolyte disorders*, ed 3. Boston, 1992, Little, Brown p. 198.

VI-2 DIFFERENTIAL DIAGNOSIS OF METABOLIC ACIDOSIS WITH INCREASED ANION GAP

I. Increased acid production
    A. Diabetic ketoacidosis
    B. Alcoholic ketoacidosis
    C. Starvation ketoacidosis
    D. Lactic acidosis
        1. Secondary to hypotension, hypovolemia, hypoxemia
        2. Secondary to drugs and toxins
        3. Enzyme defects
    E. Poisons and drug toxicity
        1. Salicylates
        2. Methanol
        3. Ethylene glycol
        4. Paraldehyde
    F. Hyperosmolar hyperglycemic nonketotic coma
II. Renal failure
    A. Acute renal failure
    B. Chronic renal failure

Modified from: Levinsky N. In Braunwald E, Isselbacher KJ, Petersdorf RG, Wilson JD, Martin J, Fauci AS, Root RK, editors: *Harrison's principles of internal medicine*, ed 12. New York, 1991, McGraw-Hill, p. 291.

VI-3 DIFFERENTIAL DIAGNOSIS OF METABOLIC ACIDOSIS WITH NORMAL ANION GAP (HYPERCHLOREMIC ACIDOSIS)

I. Renal tubular acidosis
II. Uremic acidosis (early)
III. Intestinal loss of bicarbonate or organic acid anions
   A. Diarrhea
   B. Pancreatic fistula
IV. Ureteroenterostomy
V. Drugs
   A. Acetazolamide
   B. Sulfamylon
   C. Cholestyramine
   D. Acidifying agents: NH_4Cl, oral $CaCl_2$, arginine-HCl, lysine-HCl
   E. Aldactone (in patients with cirrhosis)
VI. Rapid IV hydration
VII. Correction of respiratory alkalosis
VIII. Hyperalimentation

Modified from: Emmett M, Narins RG. Clinical use of the anion gap. *Medicine* 56:38, 1977.

VI-4 DIFFERENTIAL DIAGNOSIS OF A LOW ANION GAP

I. Reduced concentration of unmeasured anions
   A. Dilution
   B. Hypoalbuminemia
II. Increased unmeasured cations
   A. Paraproteinemia
   B. Hypercalcemia, hypermagnesemia, trimethane (tris buffer), lithium toxicity
III. Laboratory error
   A. Systemic error:
      1. Underestimation of serum sodium secondary to severe hypernatremia or hyperviscosity
      2. Bromism
   B. Random error: falsely decreased serum sodium, falsely increased serum chloride or bicarbonate

Modified from: Oh MS, Carroll HG. Current concepts. The anion gap. *N Engl J Med* 297:814, 1977 and Emmett M, Narrins RG. Clinical use of the anion gap. *Medicine* 56:38, 1977.

VI-5 DIFFERENTIAL DIAGNOSIS OF HYPOKALEMIA

I. Inadequate dietary intake
II. Gastrointestinal losses
   A. Vomiting
   B. Diarrhea
   C. Chronic laxative abuse
III. Renal losses
   A. Diuretics
   B. Mineralocorticoid excess
      1. Primary aldosteronism
         a. Adenoma
         b. Bilateral adrenal hyperplasia
      2. Cushing's syndrome
         a. Primary adrenal disease
         b. Secondary to non-endocrine tumor
      3. Accelerated hypertension
      4. Renal vascular hypertension
      5. Renin producing tumor
      6. Adrenogenital syndrome
      7. Licorice excess
   C. Bartter's syndrome
   D. Liddie's syndrome
   E. Renal tubular acidosis
   F. Metabolic alkalosis
   G. Acute hyperventilation
   H. Starvation
   I. Ureterosigmoidostomy
   J. Antibiotics — carbenicillin, amphotericin, gentamicin
   K. Diabetic ketoacidosis
   L. Acute leukemia
IV. Cellular shift
   A. Alkalosis
   B. Periodic paralysis
   C. Barium poisoning
   D. Insulin administration

Modified from: Kunau RT, Stein JH. Disorders of hypo- and hyperkalemia. *Clin Nephrol* 7:173, 1977.

VI-6 DIFFERENTIAL DIAGNOSIS OF HYPERKALEMIA

I. Pseudohyperkalemia
   A. Improper collection of blood
   B. Hematologic disorders with increased white blood cells or platelets counts
II. Exogenous potassium load
   A. Oral or intravenous KCl
   B. Potassium containing drugs
   C. Transfusion
   D. Geophagia
III. Cellular shift of potassium
   A. Tissue damage — trauma, burns, rhabdomyolysis
   B. Destruction of tumor tissue
   C. Digitalis overdose
   D. Acidosis
   E. Hyperkalemic periodic paralysis
   F. Hyperosmolality
   G. Succinylcholine
   H. Arginine infusion
IV. Decreased renal potassium excretion
   A. Acute renal failure
   B. Chronic renal failure
   C. Potassium sparing diuretics
   D. Mineralocorticoid deficiency
      1. Addison's disease
      2. Bilateral adrenalectomy
      3. Hypoaldosteronism
         a. Hyporeninemic hypoaldosteronism
         b. Heparin therapy
         c. Specific enzyme defect
         d. Tubular unresponsiveness
   E. Congenital adrenal hyperplasia
   F. Primary defect in potassium transport
   G. Use of angiotensin converting enzyme inhibitors

Modified from: Kunau RT, Stein JH. Disorders of hypo- and hyperkalemia. *Clin Nephrol* 7:173, 1977

VI-7 DIFFERENTIAL DIAGNOSIS OF HYPERNATREMIA

I. Extrarenal water loss
   A. Gastrointestinal
      1. Infantile gastroenteritis (hypertonic dehydration)
      2. Tube feeding in semi-conscious patient — increased osmotic load
   B. Skin
      1. Insensible losses
      2. Burns
      3. Sweat
   C. Lungs — insensible loss
II. Renal water loss
   A. Acute renal failure, diuretic phase
   B. Post obstruction diuresis
   C. Diabetes insipidus
   D. Osmotic diuresis — glycosuria, urea, mannitol
III. Excessive sodium intake (without access to water)
IV. Central nervous system lesions
   A. Impairment of thirst perception
   B. Stuporous or comatose patient
V. Adrenal hyperfunction
   A. Cushing's syndrome
   B. Primary hyperaldosteronism

Modified from: Levinsky N. In Braunwald E, Isselbacher KJ, Petersdorf RG, Wilson JD, Martin J, Fauci AS, Root RK, editors: *Harrison's principles of internal medicine*, ed 12. New York, 1991, McGraw-Hill, p. 280.

VI-8 DIFFERENTIAL DIAGNOSIS OF HYPONATREMIA

I. Extracellular fluid-volume depleted
  A. Renal losses
    1. Diuretics
    2. Adrenal insufficiency
    3. Salt losing nephropathy
    4. Renal tubular acidosis with bicarbonaturia
    5. Osmotic diuresis (glucose, mannitol, urea)
  B. Extra-renal losses
    1. Vomiting
    2. Diarrhea
    3. "3rd space" (e.g. burns, pancreatitis, traumatized muscle)
II. Extracellular fluid — normal or modest excess
  A. Hypothyroidism
  B. Syndrome of inappropriate ADH secretion
  C. Pain, emotion, drugs
  D. Glucocorticoid deficiency
III. Extracellular fluid-profound excess (edema)
  A. Nephrotic syndrome
  B. Cirrhosis
  C. Congestive heart failure
  D. Renal failure (acute and chronic)
IV. Artifactual
  A. Laboratory error
  B. Hyperglycemia, hypertriglyceridemia, hyperproteinemia

Modified from: Schrier RW, Berl T. In Schrier RW, editor: *Renal and electrolyte disorders*, ed 3. Boston, 1992, Little, Brown, p. 52.

VI-9 DIFFERENTIAL DIAGNOSIS OF RENAL TUBULAR ACIDOSIS (RTA) TYPE I (DISTAL)

I. Primary
  A. Idiopathic
  B. Genetic
II. Genetically transmitted systemic diseases
  A. Marfan's syndrome
  B. Sickle cell anemia
  C. Carbonic anhydrase I deficiency
  D. Galactosemia
  E. Hereditary fructose intolerance
  F. Ehlers-Danlos syndrome
  G. Fabry's disease

VI-9 DIFFERENTIAL DIAGNOSIS OF RENAL TUBULAR ACIDOSIS (RTA) TYPE I (DISTAL) (CONTINUED)

    H. Hereditary elliptocytosis
- III. Metabolic disorders
  - A. Idiopathic hypercalciuria — sporadic and hereditary
  - B. Hyperthyroidism
  - C. Primary hyperparathyroidism
  - D. Vitamin D intoxication
  - E. Mineralocorticoid deficiency
- IV. Hypergammaglobulinemic disorders
  - A. Amyloidosis
  - B. Idiopathic hyperglobulinemia
  - C. Hyperglobulinemic purpura
  - D. Cryoglobulinemia
- V. Medullary sponge kidney
- VI. Hepatic cirrhosis
- VII. Wilson's disease
- VIII. Drug induced
  - A. Amphotericin B
  - B. Vitamin D
  - C. Lithium
  - D. Toluene
  - E. Cyclamate
  - F. Analgesics
  - G. Amiloride
  - H. Glue
  - I. Balkan nephropathy
- IX. Pyelonephritis
- X. Leprosy
- XI. Renal transplantation
- XII. Obstructive nephropathy
- XIII. Autoimmune disorders
  - A. Sjögren's syndrome
  - B. Thyroiditis
  - C. Pulmonary fibrosis
  - D. Primary biliary cirrhosis
  - E. Systemic lupus erythematosus
  - F. Chronic active hepatitis
- XIV. Multiple myeloma
- XV. Hodgkin's disease

Modified from: Sebastian A, McSherry E, Morris R. In Brenner B, Rector F, editors: *The kidney*, vol 1. Philadelphia, 1986, W. B. Saunders, p. 482.

VI-10 DIFFERENTIAL DIAGNOSIS OF RENAL TUBULAR ACIDOSIS (RTA) TYPE II (PROXIMAL)

I. Primary
   A. Sporadic
   B. Genetic — Fanconi's syndrome
II. Inborn errors of metabolism
   A. Wilson's disease
   B. Cystinosis
   C. Others: Tyrosinosis, Lowe's syndrome, hereditary fructose intolerance, pyruvate carboxylase deficiency, galactosemia, glycogen storage disease (Type II)
III. Metabolic disorders
   A. Vitamin D deficiency
   B. Primary or secondary hyperparathyroidism
   C. Pseudo-vitamin D deficiency
IV. Disorders of protein metabolism
   A. Nephrotic syndrome
   B. Multiple myeloma
   C. Sjögren's syndrome
   D. Amyloidosis
   E. Other dysproteinemias
V. Medullary cystic disease
VI. Renal transplantation
VII. Drugs: outdated tetracycline, 6-mercaptopurine, streptozotocin, toluene, sulfonamide, sulfamylon, acetazolamide
VIII. Heavy metals: lead, cadmium, mercury

VI-11 DIFFERENTIAL DIAGNOSIS OF RENAL TUBULAR ACIDOSIS (RTA) TYPE IV

I. Aldosterone deficiency
   A. Combined deficiency of aldosterone and adrenal glucocorticoid hormones
      1. Addison's disease
      2. Bilateral adrenalectomy
      3. Inherited impairment of steroidogenesis: 21-hydroxylase deficiency ("congenital adrenal hyperplasia")
   B. Selective deficiency of aldosterone
      1. Inherited impairment of aldosterone biosynthesis: corticosterone methyl oxidase deficiency
      2. Secondary to deficient renin secretion
         a. Diabetic nephropathy
         b. Chronic tubulointerstitial disease with glomerular insufficiency
         c. Indomethacin administration
      3. Chronic idiopathic hypoaldosteronism in adults and children

II. Pseudohypoaldosteronism (attenuated renal response to aldosterone with secondary hyperreninemia and hyperaldosteronism)
   A. Classic pseudohypoaldosteronism of infancy
   B. Chronic tubulointerstitial disease with glomerular insufficiency "salt-wasting nephritis"
   C. Drugs: spironolactone; amiloride; triamterene

III. Attenuated renal response to aldosterone + aldosterone deficiency
   A. Selective tubule dysfunction with impaired renin secretion
   B. Chronic tubulointerstitial disease with glomerular insufficiency
      1. Associated deficient renin secretion
      2. Renin status uncertain
   C. Renal transplantation with deficient renin secretion
   D. Lupus nephritis with deficient renin secretion

IV. Uncertain pathophysiology
   A. Chronic pyelonephritis
   B. Lupus nephritis
   C. Renal transplantation
   D. Acute glomerulonephritis
   E. Renal amyloidosis

Reference: Sebastian, et. al. *Am J Med* 72:301, 1982.

VI-12 DIFFERENTIAL DIAGNOSIS OF PARENCHYMAL RENAL DISEASES CAUSING ACUTE RENAL FAILURE

I. Acute glomerulonephritis
   A. Acute poststreptococcal glomerulonephritis
   B. Systemic lupus erythematosus
   C. Bacterial endocarditis
   D. Goodpasture's syndrome
   E. Schönlein-Henoch purpura
   G. Hypersensitivity angiitis
   H. AIDS

II. Bilateral cortical necrosis
   A. Obstetrical accidents
   B. Gram-negative septicemia
   C. Ischemia
   D. Hyperacute allograft rejection
   E. Gastroenteritis (children)

III. Bilateral papillary necrosis
   A. Analgesic abuse
   B. Sickle cell disease
   C. Diabetes mellitus

IV. Diseases of tubules and/or interstitium
   A. Acute pyelonephritis
   B. Acute allergic interstitial nephritis
   C. Hypokalemic nephropathy
   D. Hypercalcemia
   E. Acute uric acid nephropathy
   F. Myeloma of the kidney

V. Diseases of the renal vasculature
   A. Renal artery occlusion
   B. Renal vein thrombosis
   C. Accelerated hypertension
   D. Accelerated scleroderma

VI. Acute nephrotoxic and/or postischemic renal failure

Modified from: Finn WF. In Earley LE, Gottschalk CW, editors: *Straus and Welt's diseases of the kidney,* ed 3. Boston, 1979, Little, Brown 1979, p. 168.

VI-13 DIFFERENTIAL DIAGNOSIS OF ACUTE DETERIORATION IN RENAL FUNCTION

I. Prerenal failure
   A. Hypovolemia from any cause
   B. Cardiovascular failure

II. Postrenal failure
   A. Extrarenal obstruction

VI-13 DIFFERENTIAL DIAGNOSIS OF ACUTE DETERIORATION IN RENAL FUNCTION (CONTINUED)

      1. Urethral occlusion or stricture
      2. Bladder, pelvic, prostatic, or retroperitoneal neoplasms
      3. Prostatism
      4. Surgical accident
      5. Calculi
      6. Pus
      7. Blood clots
      8. Sloughed papillae
  B. Intrarenal obstruction by crystals
  C. Bladder rupture

III. Renal disease
  A. Vascular
      1. Vasculitis
      2. Malignant hypertension
      3. Thrombotic thrombocytopenic purpura
      4. Scleroderma
      5. Arterial or venous occlusion
  B. Glomerulonephritis
  C. Interstitial nephritis

IV. Acute tubular necrosis
  A. Postischemic
  B. Pigment induced
      1. Hemolysis
      2. Rhabdomyolysis
  C. Toxin induced
      1. Antibiotics
      2. Contrast material
      3. Anesthetics
      4. Heavy metals
      5. Organic solvents
      6. Nonsteroidal anti-inflammatory agents
  D. Pregnancy-related
      1. Septic abortion
      2. Uterine hemorrhage
      3. Eclampsia
  E. Hypercalcemia
  F. Pyelonephritis

Modified from: Anderson R, Schrier R. In Braunwald E, Isselbacher KJ, Petersdorf RG, Wilson JD, Martin J, Fauci AS, Root RK, editors: *Harrison's principles of internal medicine*, ed 12. New York, 1991, McGraw-Hill, p. 1143.

VI-14 DIFFERENTIAL DIAGNOSIS OF COMMON MECHANICAL CAUSES OF URINARY TRACT OBSTRUCTION

Ureter*	Bladder outlet†	Urethra†
I. Congenital		
Ureteropelvic junction narrowing or obstruction	Bladder neck obstruction	Posterior urethral valves
Ureterovesical junction narrowing or obstruction	Ureterocele	Anterior urethral valves
Ureterocele		Stricture
Retrocaval ureter		Meatal stenosis
		Phimosis
II. Acquired intrinsic defects		
Calculi	Benign prostatic hypertrophy	Stricture
Inflammation	Cancer of prostate	Tumor
Trauma	Cancer of bladder	Calculi
Sloughed papillae	Calculi	Trauma
Tumor	Diabetic neuropathy	Phimosis
Blood clots	Spinal cord disease	
Uric acid crystals		

VI-14 DIFFERENTIAL DIAGNOSIS OF COMMON MECHANICAL CAUSES OF URINARY TRACT OBSTRUCTION (CONTINUED)

Ureter*	Bladder outlet†	Urethra†
III. Acquired extrinsic defects		
Pregnant uterus	Carcinoma of cervix, colon	Trauma
Retroperitoneal fibrosis		
Aortic aneurysm		
Uterine leiomyomata		
Carcinoma of uterus, prostate, bladder, colon, rectum		
Retroperitoneal lymphoma		
Accidental surgical ligation		

*Lesions are typically associated with unilateral obstruction.
†Lesions are typically associated with bilateral obstruction.

Adapted from: Brenner B, Milford EL, Seifter JL. In Braunwald E, Isselbacher KJ, Petersdorf RG, Wilson JD, Martin J, Fauci AS, Root RK, editors: *Harrison's principles of internal medicine*, ed 12. New York, 1991, McGraw-Hill, p. 1206.

VI-15 MAJOR NEPHROTOXINS

I. Exogenous
- A. Metals (Hg, Au, Ag, Ar, Pb, Cd, Ur, Li)
- B. Solvents (halogenated hydrocarbons)
- C. Diagnostic agents (contrast agents)
- D. Therapeutic agents
  1. Antibiotics (aminoglycosides, amphotericin B, sulfas, tetraycyclines, penicillins, pentamidine, foscarnet)
  2. Analgesics (phenacetin, ASA, NSAIDs)
  3. Anesthetics (methoxyflurane)
  4. Hormones (vitamin D)
  5. Antineoplastics (methotrexate, cis-platinum, cyclophosphamide)
  6. Radiation
  7. Immunosuppressive agents (cyclosporine)
- E. Miscellaneous (venoms, mushrooms, fluoride, ethylene glycol)

II. Endogenous
- A. Uric acid
- B. Oxalate
- C. Pigments (myoglobin, hemoglobin)
- D. Light chain disease
- E. Hormones (PTH)
- F. Calcium

VI-16 DIFFERENTIATION OF DEHYDRATION AND ACUTE TUBULAR INJURY AS A CAUSE OF OLIGURIA

	U_{osm} (mEq)	U_{Na}	U/P creatinine	Renal failure index $\left(\dfrac{U_{Na}}{U/P\ creatinine}\right)$	Fractional excretion Na $\left(\dfrac{U/P_{Na}}{U/P\ creatinine} \times 100\right)$	Hippuran scan	Response to fluid challenge with increased urine output	Beta$_2$ Microglobulin (mg/24hr)
Dehydration	>500	< 20	> 14:1	< 1	< 1	Kidneys well visualized	(+)	< 1.0
Acute tubular necrosis	< 350	> 30	> 14:1	> 1	> 1	Kidney poorly visualized or not at all	(−)	> 50.0

VI-17 DIFFERENTIAL DIAGNOSIS OF ACUTE GLOMERULONEPHRITIS

I. Infectious diseases
   A. Poststreptococcal glomerulonephritis
   B. Nonpoststreptococcal glomerulonephritis
      1. Bacterial: Infective endocarditis, "shunt nephritis," sepsis, pneumococcal pneumonia, typhoid fever, secondary syphilis, meningococcemia
      2. Viral: Hepatitis B, infectious mononucleosis, mumps, measles, varicella, vaccinia, echovirus, and coxsackievirus
      3. Parasitic: Malaria, toxoplasmosis
II. Multisystem diseases: Systemic lupus erythematosus, vasculitis, Schönlein-Henoch purpura, Goodpasture's syndrome
III. Primary glomerular diseases: Membranoproliferative glomerulonephritis, Berger's disease, "pure" mesangial proliferative glomerulonephritis
IV. Miscellaneous; Guillain-Barré syndrome, irradiation of Wilms' tumor, self-administered diphtheria-pertussis-tetanus vaccine, serum sickness

Adapted from: Glasslock R, Brenner R. In Braunwald E, Isselbacher KJ, Petersdorf RG, Wilson JD, Martin J, Fauci AS, Root RK, editors: *Harrison's principles of internal medicine*, ed 12. New York, 1991, McGraw-Hill, p. 1170.

VI-18 DIFFERENTIAL DIAGNOSIS OF THE NEPHROTIC SYNDROME

I. Primary glomerular disease
   A. Minimal change disease
   B. Focal and segmental glomerulosclerosis
   C. Mesangial proliferative glomerulonephritis
   D. Membranous glomerulopathy
   E. Membranoproliferative glomerulonephritis
   F. Crescentic glomerulonephritis
II. Secondary to other diseases
   A. Infections
      1. Poststreptococcal glomerulonephritis
      2. Endocarditis
      3. Hepatitis B
      4. Syphilis
      5. Leprosy
      6. "Shunt nephritis"
      7. Infectious mononucleosis
      8. Malaria

VI-18 DIFFERENTIAL DIAGNOSIS OF THE NEPHROTIC SYNDROME (CONTINUED)

      9. Schistosomiasis
     10. Filariasis
     11. AIDS

B. Drugs
    1. Gold
    2. Mercury
    3. Penicillamine
    4. Heroin
    5. Probenecid
    6. Captopril
    7. Anticonvulsants
    8. Antivenoms and antitoxins
    9. Contrast media
   10. Nonsteroidal anti-inflammatory agents

C. Neoplasms

D. Multisystem disease
    1. Systemic lupus erythematosus
    2. Schönlein-Henoch purpura
    3. Vasculitis
    4. Goodpasture's syndrome
    5. Dermatomyositis
    6. Dermatitis herpetiformis
    7. Amyloidosis
    8. Sarcoidosis
    9. Sjögren's syndrome
   10. Rheumatoid arthritis
   11. Polyarteritis nodosum

E. Heredofamilial
    1. Diabetes mellitus
    2. Alport's syndrome
    3. Myxedema
    4. Fabry's disease
    5. Nail-patella syndrome
    6. Lipodystrophy
    7. Congenital nephrotic syndrome

F. Miscellaneous
    1. Preeclamptic toxemia
    2. Thyroiditis
    3. Myxedema
    4. Malignant obesity
    5. Renovascular hypertension
    6. Chronic interstitial nephritis with vesicoureteral reflux
    7. Chronic allograft rejection
    8. Bee stings

VI-18 DIFFERENTIAL DIAGNOSIS OF THE NEPHROTIC SYNDROME (CONTINUED)

Modified from: Glassock R, Brenner R. In Braunwald E, Isselbacher KJ, Petersdorf RG, Wilson JD, Martin J, Fauci AS, Root RK, editors: *Harrison's principles of internal medicine*, ed 12. New York, 1991, McGraw-Hill, p. 1175.

VI-19 DIFFERENTIAL DIAGNOSIS OF TUBULOINTERSTITIAL DISEASE OF THE KIDNEY

I. Toxins
  A. Exogenous toxins
    1. Analgesic nephropathy
    2. Lead nephropathy
    3. Miscellaneous nephrotoxins (e.g., antibiotics, cyclosporine, radiographic contrast media, heavy metals)
  B. Metabolic toxins
    1. Acute uric acid nephropathy
    2. Gouty nephropathy
    3. Hypercalcemic nephropathy
    4. Hypokalemic nephropathy
    5. Miscellaneous metabolic toxins (e.g., hyperoxaluria, cystinosis, Fabry's disease)
II. Neoplasia
  A. Lymphoma
  B. Leukemia
  C. Multiple myeloma
III. Immune disorders
  A. Hypersensitivity nephropathy
  B. Sjögren's syndrome
  C. Amyloidosis
  D. Transplant rejection
  E. Tubulointerstitial abnormalities associated with glomerulonephritis
  F. AIDS
IV. Vascular disorders
  A. Arteriolar nephrosclerosis
  B. Atheroembolic disease
  C. Sickle-cell nephropathy
  D. Acute tubular necrosis
V. Hereditary renal diseases
  A. Hereditary nephritis (Alport's syndrome)
  B. Medullary cystic disease
  C. Medullary sponge kidney

VI-19 DIFFERENTIAL DIAGNOSIS OF TUBULOINTERSTITIAL DISEASE OF THE KIDNEY (CONTINUED)

     D. Polycystic kidney disease
- VI. Infectious injury
  - A. Acute pyelonephritis
  - B. Chronic pyelonephritis
- VII. Miscellaneous disorders
  - A. Chronic urinary tract obstruction
  - B. Radiation nephritis
  - C. Balkan nephropathy
  - D. Vesicoureteral reflux

Adapted from: Brenner B, Hosteter T. In Braunwald E, Isselbacher KJ, Petersdorf RG, Wilson JD, Martin J, Fauci AS, Root RK, editors: *Harrison's principles of internal medicine*, ed 12. New York, 1991, McGraw-Hill, p. 1187.

VI-20 DIFFERENTIAL DIAGNOSIS OF NEPHROGENIC DIABETES INSIPIDUS

- I. Congenital/familial
- II. Renal disease
  - A. Postobstructive uropathy
  - B. Polycystic disease
  - C. Medullary cystic disease
  - D. Pyelonephritis
  - E. Far-advanced renal failure
- III. Electrolyte disorders
  - A. Hypokalemia
  - B. Hypercalcemia
- IV. Drugs
  - A. Alcohol
  - B. Phenytoin
  - C. Lithium
  - D. Demeclocycline
  - E. Acetohexamide
  - F. Tolazamide
  - G. Glyburide
  - H. Propoxyphene
  - I. Amphotericin
  - J. Methoxyflurane
  - K. Norepinephrine
  - L. Vinblastine
  - M. Cisplatinum
  - N. Colchicine

VI-20 DIFFERENTIAL DIAGNOSIS OF NEPHROGENIC DIABETES INSIPIDUS (CONTINUED)

    O. Gentamicin
    P. Methicillin
    Q. Isophosphamide
    R. Contrast medium
    S. Osmotic diuretics
    T. Furosemide and ethacrynic acid
    U. Foscarnet
  V. Systemic diseases
    A. Sickle cell disease
    B. Multiple myeloma
    C. Amyloidosis
    D. Sjögren's syndrome
    E. Sarcoidosis
  VI. Dietary abnormalities
    A. Excessive water intake
    B. Decreased sodium chloride intake
    C. Decreased protein intake
  VII. Pregnancy

Adapted from: Berl T, Schrier RW. In Schrier RW, editor: *Renal and electrolyte disorders*, ed 3. Boston, 1992, Little, Brown p. 37.

VI-21 DIFFERENTIAL DIAGNOSIS OF CENTRAL DIABETES INSIPIDUS

  I. Idiopathic
    A. Sporadic
    B. Familial
  II. Head trauma
  III. Neurosurgical procedures
  IV. Neoplasms
    A. Craniopharyngioma
    B. Meningitis
    C. Metastatic (e.g., breast cancer)
  V. Lymphoma/leukemia
  VI. Infection and granulomatous disease
    A. Encephalitis
    B. Meningitis
    C. Tuberculosis
    D. Syphilis
    E. Sarcoidosis
    F. Eosinophilic granuloma

VI-21 DIFFERENTIAL DIAGNOSIS OF CENTRAL DIABETES INSIPIDUS (CONTINUED)

    VII. Vascular accidents
        A. Thrombosis
        B. Hemorrhage
        C. Sheehan's syndrome
   VIII. Histiocytosis

Modified from: Oliver R, Jamison R. Diabetes insipidus: a physiologic approach. *Postgraduate Medicine* 68:120, 1980.

VI-22 DIFFERENTIAL DIAGNOSIS OF HYPERURICEMIA

    I. Overproduction of uric acid
        A. Primary gout
        B. Myeloproliferative disorders
        C. Lymphoma
        D. Hemoglobinopathies
        E. Hemolytic anemia
        F. Psoriasis
        G. Cancer chemotherapy
    II. Underexcretion of uric acid
        A. Chronic renal failure
        B. Lead nephropathy (saturnine gout)
        C. Drugs (diuretics except spironolactone) ethambutol; low-dose aspirin
        D. Lactic acidosis (alcoholism, preeclampsia)
        E. Ketosis (diabetic, starvation)
        F. Hyperparathyroidism
        G. Hypertension
    III. Overproduction and underexcretion of uric acid: Glycogen storage disease, Type I
    IV. Mechanism unknown
        A. Sarcoidosis
        B. Obesity
        C. Hypoparathyroidism
        D. Paget's disease
        E. Down's syndrome

Adapted from: Beary JF, Scarpa NP. Manual of rheumatology and outpatient orthopedics, ed 2. Boston, 1987, Little, Brown, p. 153.

VI-23 DIFFERENTIAL DIAGNOSIS OF NEPHROLITHIASIS

    I. Calcium stones
        A. Idiopathic hypercalciuria
        B. Hyperuricosuria
        C. Primary hyperparathyroidism
        D. Distal renal tubular acidosis (RTA)
        E. Hyperoxaluria
           1. Intestinal hyperoxaluria
           2. Hereditary
        F. Idiopathic stone disease
    II. Uric acid stones
        A. Gout
        B. Idiopathic
        C. Dehydration
        D. Lesch-Nyhan syndrome
        E. Neoplasm
    III. Cystine stones (hereditary)
    IV. Struvite stones (infection)

Modified from: Coe F, Favus M. In Braunwald E, Isselbacher KJ, Petersdorf RG, Wilson JD, Martin J, Fauci AS, Root RK, editors: *Harrison's principles of internal medicine*, ed 12. New York, 1991, McGraw-Hill, p. 1203.

VI-24 DIFFERENTIAL DIAGNOSIS OF HYPOURICEMIA

    I. Decreased production
        A. Congenital xanthine oxidase deficiency
        B. Liver disease
        C. Allopurinol administration
        D. Low PP-ribose-P synthetase activity
    II. Increased excretion
        A. "Isolated" defect in renal transport of uric acid
           1. Idiopathic
           2. Neoplastic diseases
           3. Liver disease
        B. Generalized defect in renal tubular transport (Fanconi's syndrome)
           1. Idiopathic
           2. Wilson's disease
           3. Cystinosis
           4. Multiple myeloma
           5. Heavy metals
           6. Type I glycogen storage disease
           7. Galactosemia
           8. Hereditary fructose intolerance

VI-24 DIFFERENTIAL DIAGNOSIS OF HYPOURICEMIA (CONTINUED)

9. Outdated tetracyclines
10. Bronchogenic carcinoma and other neoplasms
11. Liver disease and alcoholism

C. Drugs
1. Acetoheximide
2. Azauridine
3. Benzbromarone
4. Benziodarone
5. Calcium ipodate
6. Chlorprothixene
7. Cinchophen
8. Citrate
9. Dicumarol
10. Diflumidone
11. Estrogens
12. Ethyl biscoumacetate
13. Ethyl p-chlorophenoxyisobutyric acid
14. Glyceryl guaiacolate
15. Glycine
16. Glycopyrrolate
17. Halofenate
18. Iodopyracet
19. Iopanoic acid
20. Meglumine iodipamide
21. p-Nitrophenylbutazone
22. Orotic acid
23. Outdated tetracycline
24. Phenolsulfonphthalein
25. Phenylbutazone
26. Phenylindanedione
27. Probenecid
28. Salicylates
29. Sodium diatrizoate
30. Sulfaethylthiadiazole
31. Sulfinpyrazone
32. W 2354
33. Zoxazolamine

III. Mechanism unknown
A. Pernicious anemia
B. Acute intermittent porphyria

Adapted from: Wyngaarden J, Kelley Wm. *Gout and urate metabolism.* New York, 1976, Grune & Stratton, p. 412.

VI-25 RENAL COMPLICATIONS OF NEOPLASMS

   I. Glomerulonephritis, with or without nephrotic syndrome
  II. Obstructive uropathy
      A. Tubular precipitation syndromes
          1. Uric acid nephropathy
          2. Hypercalcemic nephropathy
          3. Paraproteinuric syndromes
              a. Multiple myeloma
              b. Other (monoclonal gammopathy, lysozymuria, mucoproteins, proteolytic products)
      B. Obstruction of the ureters, bladder, and urethra
 III. Direct invasion by malignant process
      A. Primary renal tumors
      B. Metastatic infiltration
  IV. Treatment-related nephropathies
      A. Radiation nephropathy
      B. Drug-induced nephrotoxicity
          1. Cytotoxic drugs
          2. Drugs used in supportive care
              a. Antibiotics
              b. Analgesics
          3. Immunotherapy
   V. Miscellaneous
      A. Disseminated intravascular coagulation
      B. Amyloidosis
      C. Electrolyte abnormalities

Adapted from: Fer, et al. *Amer J Med* 71:705, 1981.

VI-26 CONDITIONS LEADING TO GENERALIZED EDEMA

I. Kidney diseases
   A. Acute glomerulonephritis
   B. Nephrotic syndrome
   C. Acute renal failure
   D. Chronic renal failure
II. Heart failure
III. Liver diseases
   A. Cirrhosis
   B. Obstruction of hepatic venous outflow
IV. Conditions confined to women
   A. Normal pregnancy
   B. Toxemia of pregnancy
   C. Idiopathic edema
V. Vascular diseases
   A. Arteriovenous fistulas
   B. Obstruction of inferior or superior vena cava
VI. Endocrine disorders
   A. Hypothyroidism
   B. Mineralocorticoid excess
   C. Diabetes mellitus
VII. Iatrogenic disorders
   A. Drugs — oral contraceptives, estrogens, antihypertensives
   B. Excessive intravenous infusion of saline solutions
VIII. Miscellaneous
   A. Chronic hypokalemia
   B. Chronic anemia
   C. Nutritional edema
   D. Capillary leak syndrome
   E. Filariasis
   F. High-altitude edema

Modified from: Levy M, Seely JF. In Brenner and Rector, editors: *The kidney*, ed 2. Philadelphia, 1981, W. B. Saunders, 1981, p. 726.

VI-27 CLINICAL SPECTRUM OF ABNORMALITIES IN UREMIA

I. Fluid and electrolyte disturbances
   A. Volume expansion and contraction
   B. Hypernatremia and hyponatremia
   C. Hyperkalemia and hypokalemia
   D. Metabolic acidosis
   E. Hyperphosphatemia and hypophosphatemia
   F. Hypocalcemia

II. Endocrine-metabolic disturbances
   A. Renal osteodystrophy
   B. Secondary hyperparathyroidism
   C. Carbohydrate intolerance
   D. Hyperuricemia
   E. Hypothermia
   F. Hypertriglyceridemia
   G. Protein-calorie malnutrition
   H. Impaired growth and development
   I. Infertility and sexual dysfunction
   J. Amenorrhea

III. Neuromuscular disturbances
   A. Fatigue
   B. Sleep disorders
   C. Headache
   D. Impaired mentation
   E. Lethargy
   F. Asterixis
   G. Muscular irritability
   H. Peripheral neuropathy
   I. Restless legs syndrome
   J. Paralysis
   K. Myoclonus
   L. Seizures
   M. Coma
   N. Muscle cramps
   O. Dialysis disequilibrium syndrome
   P. Dialysis dementia
   Q. Myopathy

IV. Cardiovascular and pulmonary disturbances
   A. Arterial hypertension
   B. Congestive heart failure
   C. Pericarditis
   D. Cardiomyopathy
   E. Uremic lung
   F. Accelerated atherosclerosis
   G. Hypotension and arrhythmias

VI-27 CLINICAL SPECTRUM OF ABNORMALITIES IN UREMIA (CONTINUED)

V. Dermatologic disturbances
   A. Pallor
   B. Hyperpigmentation
   C. Pruritus
   D. Ecchymoses
   E. Uremic frost
VI. Gastrointestinal disturbances
   A. Anorexia
   B. Nausea and vomiting
   C. Uremic fetor
   D. Gastroenteritis
   E. Peptic ulcer
   F. GI bleeding
   G. Hepatitis
   H. Refractory ascites
   I. Peritonitis
VII. Hematologic and immunologic disturbances
   A. Normocytic, normochromic anemia
   B. Microcytic (aluminum-induced) anemia
   C. Lymphocytopenia
   D. Bleeding diathesis
   E. Increased susceptibility to infection
   F. Splenomegaly and hypersplenism
   G. Leukopenia
   H. Hypocomplementemia

Modified from: Brenner BM. In Braunwald E, Isselbacher KJ, Petersdorf RG, Wilson JD, Martin J, Fauci AS, Root RK, editors: *Harrison's principles of internal medicine*, ed 12. New York, 1991, McGraw-Hill, p. 1153.

VI-28 DIFFERENTIAL DIAGNOSIS OF RESPIRATORY ACIDOSIS

I. Acute respiratory acidosis
   A. Neuromuscular abnormalities
      1. Brain stem injury
      2. High cord injury
      3. Guillain-Barré syndrome
      4. Myasthenia gravis
      5. Botulism
      6. Narcotic, sedative or tranquilizer overdose
   B. Airway obstruction
      1. Foreign body
      2. Aspiration of vomitus
      3. Laryngeal edema
      4. Severe bronchospasm
   C. Thoracic-pulmonary disorders
      1. Flail chest
      2. Pneumothorax
      3. Severe pneumonia
      4. Smoke inhalation
      5. Severe pulmonary edema
   D. Massive pulmonary embolism
   E. Respirator controlled ventilation
      1. Inadequate frequency, tidal volume settings
      2. Large dead space
      3. Total parenteral nutrition
II. Chronic respiratory acidosis
   A. Neuromuscular abnormalities
      1. Chronic narcotic or sedative ingestion
      2. Primary hypoventilation
      3. Pickwickian syndrome
      4. Poliomyelitis
      5. Diaphragmatic paralysis
   B. Thoracic-pulmonary disorders
      1. Chronic obstructive airway disease
      2. Kyphoscoliosis
      3. End-stage interstitial pulmonary disease

Modified from: Kaehny WG. In Schrier RW, editor: *Renal and electrolyte disorders*, ed 3. Boston, 1992, Little, Brown, p. 215.

VI-29 DIFFERENTIAL DIAGNOSIS OF RESPIRATORY ALKALOSIS

I. Central stimulation of respiration
   A. Anxiety
   B. Head trauma
   C. Brain tumors or vascular accidents
   D. Salicylates
   E. Fever
   F. Pain
   G. Pregnancy
II. Peripheral stimulation of respiration
   A. Pulmonary emboli
   B. Congestive heart failure
   C. Interstitial lung diseases
   D. Pneumonia
   E. "Stiff lungs" without hypoxemia
   F. Altitude
   G. Asthma
III. Uncertain
   A. Hepatic insufficiency
   B. Gram-negative septicemia
IV. Mechanical or voluntary hyperventilation

Modified from: Kaehny WG. In Schrier RW, editor: *Renal and electrolyte disorders*, ed 3. Boston, 1992, Little, Brown, p. 221.

VI-30 RULES OF THUMB FOR BEDSIDE INTERPRETATION OF ACID-BASE DISORDERS

Metabolic acidosis	$PaCO_2$ should fall by 1.0 to 1.5 x the fall in plasma HCO_3 concentration
Metabolic alkalosis	$PaCO_2$ should rise by 0.24 to 1.0 x the rise in plasma HCO_3 concentration
Acute respiratory acidosis	Plasma HCO_3 concentration should rise by about 1 mmole/L for each 10 mmHg increment in $PaCO_2$ ($\pm$3 mmoles/L)
Chronic respiratory acidosis	Plasma HCO_3 concentration should rise about 4 mmoles/L for each 10 mmHg increment in $PaCO_2$ ($\pm$4 mmoles/L)
Acute respiratory alkalosis	Plasma HCO_3 concentration should fall by about 1-3 mmoles/L for each 10 mmHg decrement in the $PaCO_2$, usually not to less than 18 mmoles/L
Chronic respiratory alkalosis	Plasma HCO_3 concentration should fall by about 2-5 mmoles/L per 10 mmHg decrement in $PaCO_2$ but usually not to less than 14 mmoles/L

Adapted from: Kaehny WG, Shapiro JI. In Schrier RW, editor: *Renal and electrolyte disorders*, ed 3. Boston, 1992, Little, Brown, p. 167.

VI-31 COMPLICATIONS OF DIALYSIS

Access	Dialysis procedure
Infection	Hemorrhage
Thrombosis	Hypotension
Vascular compromise	Cardiac ischemia
High-output CHF	Cramps, nausea, vomiting
Carpal tunnel syndrome	Seizures
Recirculation of blood flow	Hypoventilation, hypoxemia
	Anticoagulation
	Air embolism
	Hemolysis

From: Carpenter CB, Lazarus JM. In Braunwald E, Isselbacher KJ, Petersdorf RG, Wilson JD, Martin J, Fauci AS, Root RK, editors: *Harrison's principles of internal medicine*, ed 12. New York, 1991, McGraw-Hill, p. 388.

VI-32 CAUSES OF HEMATURIA

I. Glomerular causes of hematuria
  A. Proliferative diseases of the glomerulus
    1. Primary
      a. IgA nephropathy (Berger's disease)
      b. Poststreptococcal glomerulonephritis
      c. Membranoproliferative glomerulonephritis
      d. Idiopathic rapidly progressive glomerulonephritis
      e. Fibrillary glomerulonephritis
    2. Secondary (Associated with Multisystem Diseases)
      a. Postinfectious glomerulonephritis
      b. Schölein-Henoch purpura
      c. Systemic lupus erythematosus
      d. Goodpasture's syndrome
      e. Vasculitis
      f. Essential mixed cryoglobulinemia
  B. Nonproliferative diseases of the glomerulus
    1. Membranous glomerulopathy
    2. Focal and segmental glomerulosclerosis
    3. Diabetic glomerulosclerosis
  C. Familiar diseases of the glomerulus
    1. Alport's syndrome
    2. Thin basement membrane diseases
    3. Fabry's disease
    4. Nail-patella syndrome
II. Nonglomular renal parenchymal causes of hematuria
  A. Neoplasms
    1. Renal cell carcinoma
    2. Wilms's tumor
    3. Benign cyst
  B. Vascular
    1. Renal infarct
    2. Renal vein thrombosis
    3. Malignant hypertension
    4. Arteriovenous malformation
    5. Papillary necrosis
    6. Loin-pain hematuria syndrome
  C. Metabolic
    1. Hypercalciuria
    2. Hyperuricosuria
  D. Familial
    1. Polycystic kidney diseases
      a. Medullary sponge kidney
  E. Drugs
    1. Anticoagulants (heparin, coumadin)
    2. Drug-induced acute interstitial nephritis
  F. Trauma

VI-32 CAUSES OF HEMATURIA (CONTINUED)

III. Extrarenal causes of hematuria

   A. Calculi

      1. Ureter, bladder, prostate

   B. Neoplasms

      1. Transitional cell carcinoma (pelvis, ureter and bladder)

      2. Adenocarcinoma and benign hypertrophy (prostate)

      3. Squamous cell carcinoma (urethra)

   C. Infections

      1. Acute cystitis, prostatitis, and urethritis

      2. Tuberculosis

      3. *Schistosoma haematobium*

   D. Drugs

      1. Anticoagulants (heparin; coumadin)

      2. Cyclophosphamide (hemorrhagic cystitis)

   F. Trauma

From: Lieberthal, W. *The principles and practice of nephrology*, Jacobson, H.R., Striker, G.E. and Klahr, S. (eds.), B.C. Decker Company, Philadelphia, 1991, p. 245-246.

CHAPTER VII
PULMONARY DISEASE

VII-1 DIFFERENTIAL DIAGNOSIS OF CLUBBING OF THE DIGITS

I. Pulmonary disorders
   A. Infection
      1. Bronchiectasis
      2. Lung abscess
      3. Empyema
      4. Tuberculosis (only with extensive fibrosis or abscess)
   B. Neoplasm
      1. Primary lung cancer
      2. Metastatic lung cancer
      3. Mesothelioma
   C. Pulmonary fibrosis
   D. Arteriovenous malformations
   E. Neurogenic diaphragmatic tumors
   F. Cystic fibrosis
II. Cardiac disorders
   A. Congenital cyanotic heart disease
   B. Infective endocarditis
III. Gastrointestinal disorders
   A. Ulcerative colitis
   B. Regional enteritis
   C. Hepatic cirrhosis
IV. Miscellaneous
   A. Hemiplegia

Modified from: Szidor JP and Fishman AP. In Fishman AP, editor: *Pulmonary diseases and disorders*, ed 2, vol 1. New York, 1988, McGraw-Hill, p. 318.

VII-2 DIFFERENTIAL DIAGNOSIS OF HEMOPTYSIS

I. Infections
   *A. Bronchitis, esp. chronic
   B. Bronchiectasis
   *C. Pneumonia
   D. Lung abscess
   E. Tuberculosis
   F. Fungal

II. Neoplasms
   *A. Bronchogenic carcinoma
   B. Bronchial adenoma

III. Cardiovascular disorders
   *A. Pulmonary infarction
   B. Mitral stenosis
   C. Pulmonary congestion and alveolar edema
   D. Aortic aneurysm
   E. Pulmonary arteriovenous fistula

IV. Trauma

V. Miscellaneous
   A. Foreign body
   B. Broncholith
   C. Bleeding diathesis
   D. Goodpasture's syndrome
   E. Wegener's granulomatosis

*most common

Modified from: Fishman AP. In Fishman AP, editor: *Pulmonary diseases and disorders*, ed 2, vol 1. New York, 1988, McGraw-Hill, p. 347.

VII-3 DIFFERENTIAL DIAGNOSIS OF BRONCHIECTASIS

I. Bronchopulmonary Infections
II. Bronchial Obstruction
    A. Laryngeal papillomatosis
    B. Bronchogenic carcinoma
    C. Allergic bronchopulmonary aspergillosis
    D. Chronic bronchitis
III. Congenital/Hereditary
    A. Williams-Campbell syndrome (cartilage deficiency)
    B. Mounier-Kuhn syndrome (tracheobronchomegaly)
    C. Pulmonary Sequestration
    D. Yellow-nail syndrome
    E. Immunodeficiency states
    F. Immotile cilia syndrome
    G. Kartagener's syndrome
    H. α_1-Antitrypsin deficiency
    I. Cystic fibrosis
IV. Miscellaneous
    A. Young's syndrome
    B. Recurrent aspiration

Modified from: Swartz M. In Fishman AP, editor: *Pulmonary diseases and disorders*, ed 2, vol 2. New York, 1988, McGraw-Hill, p. 1559.

VII-4 DIFFERENTIAL DIAGNOSIS OF PLEURAL EFFUSIONS

I. Transudates
   A. Congestive heart failure
   B. Nephrotic syndrome
   C. Liver conditions with ascites (hepatic hydrothorax)
   D. Peritoneal dialysis
   E. Meigs syndrome
   F. Hydronephrosis
   G. Myxedema
II. Exudates
   A. Predominant
      1. Parapneumonic
      2. Malignant
      3. Pulmonary embolic
   B. Common
      1. Tuberculosis
      2. Traumatic
      3. Abdominal disease
      4. Collagen vascular disease (esp. RA and SLE)
   C. Unusual
      1. Drug-induced (e.g., Nitrofurantoin)
      2. Asbestos
      3. Dressler's syndrome
      4. Chylothorax
      5. Uremia
      6. Radiation therapy
      7. Sarcoidosis
      8. Yellow-nail syndrome

Modified from: Kinasewitz GT, et al. In Fishman AP, editor: *Pulmonary diseases and disorders*, ed 2, vol 3. New York, 1988, McGraw-Hill, p. 2134.

VII-5 EVALUATION OF PLEURAL EFFUSIONS

	Transudate	Exudate
I. Protein		
Absolute value	< 2 g/dl	> 3 g/dl
Pleural fluid/serum ratio	< 0.5	> 0.5
II. LDH		
Absolute value	< 200 IU/L	> 200 IU/L
Pleural fluid/serum ratio	< 0.6	> 0.6
III. Glucose	> 60 mg/dl	< 60 mg/dl
IV. Leukocytes	< 1000/ml	> 1000/ml
PMNs	< 50%	> 50%
V. Erythrocytes	< 5000/ml	Variable

Modified from: Pierson D. In Braunwald E, Isselbacher KJ, Petersdorf RG, Wilson JD, Martin J, Fauci AS, Root RK, editors: *Harrison's principles of internal medicine*, ed 12. New York, 1991, McGraw-Hill, p. 1111.

VII-6 DIFFERENTIAL DIAGNOSIS OF COUGH WITH NEGATIVE CHEST X-RAY

I. Acute respiratory infections
II. Acute irritative bronchitis (inhaled or aspirated irritant)
   A. Exogenous irritants (tobacco smoke, smog, high levels of O_2, noxious gases in workplace)
   B. Mechanical irritants (foreign body, postnasal drip, gastric contents, retained bronchopulmonary secretions)
III. Postbronchitis cough syndrome
IV. Chronic bronchitis
V. Asthma
VI. Bronchiectasis
VII. Congestive heart failure
VIII. Esophageal disease which results in recurrent aspiration
   A. Esophageal reflux
   B. Achalasia
   C. Zenker's diverticulum
IX. Tracheobronchial neoplasms
   A. Primary tracheal neoplasms
   B. Secondary tracheal malignancy
   C. Bronchogenic carcinoma
   D. Bronchial adenoma
   E. Metastatic tumors
X. Nonneoplastic bronchial obstructive lesions
   A. Foreign body
   B. Broncholithiasis
   C. Bronchial stricture
   D. Extrinsic compression
XI. Cystic fibrosis
XII. Laryngeal lesions
XIII. Postnasal discharge
XIV. Psychogenic cough
XV. Pulmonary emboli

VII-7 DIFFERENTIAL DIAGNOSIS OF HILAR ENLARGEMENT

I. Unilateral
- A. Malignancy
  1. Primary bronchogenic carcinoma
  2. Metastatic lymphadenopathy
- B. Infections
  1. Tuberculosis
  2. Fungal
  3. Bacterial (occasionally)
- C. Sarcoidosis
- D. Lymph node hyperplasia
- E. Pulmonary artery enlargement
- F. Mediastinal masses

II. Bilateral
- A. Sarcoidosis
- B. Infection
  1. Tuberculosis
  2. Fungal
  3. Mononucleosis
  4. Mycoplasma
- C. Metastatic tumor
- D. Lymphoma
- E. Pneumoconioses
  1. Silicosis
  2. Berylliosis
- F. Vascular
  1. Enlargement of pulmonary arteries
     a. Pulmonary emboli
     b. Chronic cor pulmonale
  2. Enlargement of pulmonary veins
     a. Congestive heart failure
     b. Mitral stenosis

VII-8 DIFFERENTIAL DIAGNOSIS OF PNEUMOTHORAX

   I. Primary spontaneous pneumothorax
  II. Iatrogenic
 III. Traumatic
 IV. Mediastinal emphysema
  V. Pulmonary inflammation
     A. Tuberculosis
     B. Coccidioidomycosis (other fungal infections less commonly)
     C. Staphylococcal pneumonia with abscess (other bacterial pneumonias)
     D. Pneumocystis carinii pneumonia (PCP)
 VI. Rupture of cysts and bullae
VII. "Honeycomb" lungs (pulmonary microcysts)
     A. Idiopathic
     B. Cystic fibrosis
     C. Scleroderma
     D. Eosinophilic granuloma
     E. Pulmonary tuberous sclerosis
     F. Pulmonary lymphangiomatoid granulomatosis
     G. Pneumoconioses
     H. Marfan's syndrome
VIII. Catamenial pneumothorax
 IX. Miscellaneous
     A. Asthma
     B. Pulmonary infarction with cavitation
     C. Eosinophilic
     D. Pseudoxanthoma elasticum
     E. Ehlers-Danlos
     F. Pulmonary hemosiderosis
     G. Paragonimiasis
     H. Pulmonary alveolar proteinosis
     I. Hydatid lung disease
     J. Rheumatoid lung disease

VII-9 DIFFERENTIAL DIAGNOSIS OF RECURRENT PULMONARY INFECTION ASSOCIATED WITH IMMUNODEFICIENCY SYNDROMES OTHER THAN HIV-RELATED

I. Antibody (B-cell) deficiency syndromes
   A. Common, variable, acquired hypogammaglobulinemia
   B. Congenital, X-linked hypogammaglobulinemia
   C. Transient hypogammaglobulinemia of infancy
   D. Selective IgA deficiency
   E. Selective IgM deficiency
   F. Selective IgG subclass deficiency

II. Complement deficiency syndromes
   A. C'3 deficiency
   B. C'5 dysfunction

III. Phagocyte deficiency syndromes
   A. Granulocytopenia
   B. Chronic granulomatous disease
   C. Myeloperoxidase deficiency
   D. Chediak-Higashi syndrome
   E. "Lazy leukocyte" syndrome

IV. Cellular (T-cell) deficiency syndromes
   A. Congenital thymic aplasia
   B. Chronic mucocutaneous candidiasis

V. Combined antibody and cellular deficiency syndromes
   A. Severe combined immunodeficiency
   B. Ataxia-Telangiectasia
   C. Wiskott-Aldrich syndrome

Modified from: Dauber JH, et al. In Fishman AP, editor: *Pulmonary diseases and disorders*, vol 2. New York, 1980, McGraw-Hill, p. 1002.

VII-10 DIFFERENTIAL DIAGNOSIS OF EOSINOPHILIC LUNG DISEASE

I. Idiopathic
   A. Transient pulmonary eosinophilia (Loeffler's)
   B. Prolonged pulmonary eosinophilia (Carrington's)
II. Eosinophilic lung diseases of specific etiology
   A. Drug induced (i.e., nitrofurantoin and penicillin)
   B. Parasite induced
      1. Strongyloides
      2. Ancylostomiasis
      3. Tropical pulmonary eosinophilia
      4. Pulmonary larva migrans
      5. Schistosomiasis
      6. Toxocara
      7. *Necator americanus*
   C. Fungus induced
      1. Hypersensitivity bronchopulmonary aspergillosis
III. Eosinophilic lung disease associated with angiitis and/or granulomatosis
   A. Wegener's granulomatosis
   B. Allergic granulomatosis
   C. Polyarteritis nodosa
   D. Necrotizing alveolitis
   E. Necrotizing "sarcoidal" angiitis and granulomatosis

Modified from: Fraser RG, Para JA. *Diagnosis of diseases of the chest*, ed 3 vol 2. Philadelphia, 1988, W. B. Saunders, p. 1291.

VII-11 DIFFERENTIAL DIAGNOSIS OF PULMONARY INTERSTITIAL DISEASE OF KNOWN ETIOLOGY

I. Occupational /environmental agents
  A. Inorganic dusts (e.g., silica, asbestos)
  B. Organic dusts (e.g., sugar cane)
  C. Fumes
    1. Nitrogen dioxine
    2. Chlorine, ammonia, sulfur dioxide
II. Drugs
  A. Sulfonamides
  B. Bleomycin
  C. Busulfan
  D. Nitrofurantoin
  E. Gold salts
  F. Amiodarone
III. Radiation
IV. Infectious agents
  A. Viruses (influenza, CMV, varicella)
  B. Bacterial
  C. Fungal (histoplasmosis, coccidioidomycosis)
  D. Parasites (schistosomiasis, pneumocystis carinii)
V. Cardiac disease (CHF)
VI. Metabolic abnormalities

Modified from: Jackson L, Fulmer J. In Fishman AP, editor: *Pulmonary diseases and disorders*, ed 2, vol 1. New York, 1988, McGraw-Hill, p. 740.

VII-12 DIFFERENTIAL DIAGNOSIS OF PULMONARY INTERSTITIAL DISEASE OF UNKNOWN ETIOLOGY

I. Sarcoidosis
II. Collagen vascular disorders
  A. Rheumatoid lung
  B. Scleroderma
  C. Sjögren's syndrome
  D. Systemic lupus erythematosus
III. Idiopathic pulmonary fibrosis
IV. Histiocytosis X
V. Pulmonary hemorrhagic syndromes
  A. Idiopathic hemosiderosis
  B. Goodpasture's
VI. Lymphangioleiomyomatosis
VII. Ankylosing spondylitis

VII-12 DIFFERENTIAL DIAGNOSIS OF PULMONARY INTERSTITIAL DISEASE OF UNKNOWN ETIOLOGY (CONTINUED)

   VIII. Chronic eosinophilic pneumonias
      A. Hypersensitivity pneumonitis
   IX. Veno-occlusive disease
      A. Pulmonary emboli
   X. Pulmonary vasculitis

Modified from: Jackson L, Fulmer J. In Fishman AP, editor: *Pulmonary diseases and disorders*, ed 2, vol 1. New York, 1988, McGraw-Hill, p. 740.

VII-13 DIFFERENTIAL DIAGNOSIS OF RESPIRATORY FAILURE

   I. Pulmonary origin
      A. Diffuse obstructive airway disease
      B. Central airway obstruction
      C. Restrictive lung disease
      D. Adult respiratory distress syndrome
      E. Pulmonary vascular disease
         1. Pulmonary embolus
         2. Arteriovenous fistula
         3. Veno-occlusive disease
      F. Pleural and chest wall disease
         1. Pleural effusions
         2. Pleural fibrosis
         3. Pneumothorax
         4. Flail chest
         5. Fixed chest wall deformities
      G. Diaphragm muscle fatigue
      H. Metastatic tumor
      I. Infections
   II. Extrapulmonary origin
      A. Neuromuscular disease
         1. Potentiated by electrolyte abnormalities ($\downarrow$K, $\downarrow$PO$_4$)
         2. Guillain-Barré syndrome
      B. Central nervous system disease
      C. Drug suppression of respiratory center
      D. Primary hypoventilation syndromes (sleep apnea syndromes)
         1. Central type
         2. Obstructive
         3. Mixed
      E. Laryngeal obstruction
      F. Congestive heart failure

VII-14 GUIDELINES FOR WITHDRAWAL OF MECHANICAL VENTILATION

    I. An awake and alert mental state

   II. PaO_2 > 60 mm Hg, with FIO_2 ≤ 0.5

  III. PEEP ≤ 5 cm H_2O

  IV. $PaCO_2$ acceptable, with pH in the normal range

   V. Vital capacity >10-15 mg/kg

  VI. Minute ventilation <10 liters/minute; respiratory rate < 25/minute

 VII. Maximum voluntary ventilation double that of minute ventilation

VIII. Peak inspiratory pressure lower (more negative) than –25 cm H_2O

  IX. Spontaneous ventilation via T tube (with or without CPAP) for 1-4 hours with acceptable blood gases and without marked increases in respiratory rate, heart rate, or change in general status

Modified from: Woodley M, Whelan A. In Orland MJ, Saltman RJ, editors: *Manual of Medical Therapeutics* ed 27. Boston, 1992, Little, Brown p. 191.

VII-15 DIFFERENTIAL DIAGNOSIS OF ALVEOLAR HYPERVENTILATION

I. Increase in stimuli from the periphery
   A. Hypoxia
   B. Diffuse interstitial edema or disease
   C. Pulmonary emboli
   D. Pain
   E. Circulatory collapse
   F. Cooling
II. Increase in stimuli from central nervous system
   A. Anxiety
   B. Voluntary
   C. Fever
   D. Brain stem lesions
   E. Salicylates
   F. Intracranial hemorrhage
   G. Metabolic acidosis
   H. Descent from altitude
III. Unknown stimuli
   A. Cirrhosis of the liver
   B. Uremia
   C. Pregnancy
IV. Assisted ventilation

Modified from: Fishman AP. In Fishman AP, editor: *Pulmonary diseases and disorders*, ed 2, vol 1. New York, 1988, McGraw-Hill, p. 301.

248

VII-16 DIFFERENTIAL DIAGNOSIS OF CHRONIC ALVEOLAR HYPOVENTILATION

I. Functional depression of ventilatory drive
 A. Sleep
 B. Hypercapnea
 C. Metabolic alkalosis
 D. Drugs (narcotics, sedatives)
 E. Myxedema
II. Anatomic damage to respiratory neurons
 A. Bulbar poliomyelitis
 B. Encephalitis
 C. Brain-stem infarction
 D. Brain-stem neoplasm
 E. Bilateral cervical cordotomy
III. Idiopathic alveolar hypoventilation
IV. Organic depression of motor pathways (Ondine's curse)
V. Peripheral neuromuscular disorders
 A. Poliomyelitis
 B. Guillain-Barré syndrome
 C. Myasthenia gravis
 D. Muscular dystrophy
 E. Polymyositis
 F. Bilateral diaphragmatic paralysis
VI. Disorders of the chest cage
 A. Kyphoscoliosis
 B. Obesity — hypoventilation syndromes
VII. Obstruction of the upper airways
 A. Tracheal stenosis
 B. Obstructive sleep apnea

Modified from: Millman RR and Fishman AP. In Fishman AP, editor: *Pulmonary diseases and disorders*, ed 2, vol 1. New York, 1988, McGraw-Hill, p. 1335.

VII-17 SYMPTOMS AND SIGNS OBSERVED IN 327 PATIENTS WITH ANGIOGRAPHICALLY DOCUMENTED PULMONARY EMBOLI

Symptoms and signs	%
Symptoms	
Chest pain	88
Pleuritic	74
Nonpleuritic	14
Dyspnea	85
Apprehension	59
Cough	53
Hemoptysis	30
Sweats	27
Syncope	13
Signs	
Respirations >16/min.	92
Rales	58
Increased S_2P*	53
Pulse >100 min.	44
Temperature >37.8°C	43
Diaphoresis	36
Gallop	34
Phlebitis	32
Edema	24
Murmur	23
Cyanosis	19

*Increased S_2P = increase in intensity of the pulmonic component of the second heart sound.

Modified from: Bell WR, Simon TS, DeMets DL. The clinical features of submassive and massive pulmonary emboli. *Am J Med* 62:355, 1977.

VII-18 ECG CHANGES IN PULMONARY EMBOLISM

Normal sinus rhythm or sinus tachycardia	75% to 80%
Rhythm changes	20% to 25%
Premature atrial contractions	10%
Premature ventricular contractions	10%
Atrial fibrillation	5%
Conduction disturbance	10%
QRS axis changes	
Acute right shift (S_1Q_3 pattern)	15%
Right bundle branch block	8%
T changes	40%
Depressed ST segments	25%
Elevated ST segments	16%

*Significantly more common in massive embolism.

Reference: Stein PD, Dalen JE, McIntyre KM, Sasahara AA, Wenger NK, Willis PW. The electrocardiogram in acute pulmonary embolism. *Progr Cardiovasc Dis* 17:247, 1974.

VII-19 CLINICAL DISORDERS ASSOCIATED WITH THE ADULT RESPIRATORY DISTRESS SYNDROME

I. Sepsis
II. Trauma
   A. Fat emboli
   B. Lung contusion
   C. Massive blood transfusions
III. Liquid aspiration
   A. Gastric contents
   B. Fresh and salt water (drowning)
   C. Hydrocarbon fluids
IV. Drug-associated
   A. Heroin
   B. Cocaine
   C. Ethchlorvynol
   D. Aspirin
V. Inhaled toxins
   A. Smoke
   B. Corrosive chemicals (NO_2, CL_2, NH_3, phosgene)
VI. Shock of any etiology
VII. Hematologic disorders
   A. Thrombocytopenic purpura
   B. Disseminated intravascular coagulation
VIII. Metabolic
   A. Acute pancreatitis
IX. Miscellaneous
   A. Lymphangiography
   B. Re-expansion pulmonary edema
   C. Neurogenic pulmonary edema
   D. Postcardiopulmonary bypass
   E. Eclampsia
   F. Air emboli
   G. Amniotic fluid embolism
   H. Ascent to high altitude

Modified from: Matthay MA. Pathophysiology of pulmonary edema. *Clin. Chest Med.* 6:311, 1985.

VII-20 PROGNOSTIC INDICATORS IN PNEUMOCOCCAL PNEUMONIA

I. Multilobe involvement (hypoxia)
II. Metastatic sites of infection such as bone, pericardium, meningitis (positive blood cultures)
III. Immunocompromised states
   A. Hodgkin's and non-Hodgkin's lymphoma
   B. Leukemia
   C. Corticosteroid use
IV. Asplenic states (sickle cell anemia, post-splenectomy)
V. HIV infection
VI. WBC < 5000 or > 25,000
VII. Extremes of age (young & old) < 1 or > 55
VIII. Complement abnormalities
IX. Agammaglobulinemia
X. Pre-existing illnesses (chronic lung disease, diabetes mellitus)
XI. Ethanolism

VII-21 CLASSIFICATION OF LUNG ABSCESSES ACCORDING TO CAUSE

I. Necrotizing infections
   A. Pyogenic bacteria (*S. aureus*, Klebsiella, group A streptococcus, Bacteroides, Fusobacterium, anaerobic and microaerophilic cocci and streptococci, other anaerobes, Nocardia)
   B. Mycobacteria (*Mycobacterium tuberculosis*, *M. kansasii*, *Pseudomonas aeruginosa*, Legionella, *M. avium intracellulare*)
   C. Fungi (Histoplasma, Coccidioides, Aspergillus)
   D. Parasites (amoeba, lung flukes)
II. Cavitary infarction
   A. Bland embolism
   B. Septic embolism (various anaerobes, Staphylococcus, Candida)
   C. Vasculitis (Wegener's granulomatosis, polyarteritis)
III. Cavitary malignancy
   A. Primary bronchogenic carcinoma
   B. Metastatic malignancies (very uncommon)
IV. Other
   A. Infected cysts
   B. Necrotic conglomerate lesions (silicosis, coal miner's pneumoconiosis)

Modified from: Reynolds H. In Braunwald E, Isselbacher KJ, Petersdorf RG, Wilson JD, Martin J, Fauci AS, Root RK, editors: *Harrison's principles of internal medicine*, ed 12. New York, 1991, McGraw-Hill, p. 1068.

VII-22 CRITERIA FOR THE DIAGNOSIS OF ALLERGIC BRONCHOPULMONARY ASPERGILLOSIS

I. Primary
   A. Asthma
   B. Peripheral blood and sputum eosinophilia
   C. Positive immediate skin test
   D. Positive serum precipitins
   E. Elevated IgE levels
   F. Recurrent pulmonary infiltrates
   G. Central bronchiectasis on bronchograms
II. Secondary
   A. Aspergillus in sputum on repeated culture
   B. Expectoration of "brown plugs"
   C. Positive 6-8 hour delayed skin test

Note: The first six primary signs should be present for the diagnosis to be made.

Reference: Corrigan K and Kory R. Diagnosis and management of pulmonary aspergillosis. Ann Intern Med 86:405, 1977.

VII-23 SOLITARY PULMONARY NODULES

I. Differential diagnosis of a solitary pulmonary nodule*
   A. Malignant neoplasm
      1. Primary lung carcinoma or sarcoma
      2. Metastatic carcinoma or sarcoma
   B. Inflammation
      1. Granulomas
      2. Inflammatory pseudotumor
      3. Localized scar
   C. Benign neoplasms
      1. "Hamartoma"
      2. Other mesenchymal tumors
      3. Clear cell ("sugar") tumor
   D. Malformation
      1. Pulmonary sequestration
II. Common nonmalignant lesions presenting as solitary pulmonary nodules†
   A. Very common
      1. Granulomas
         a. Histoplasmoma, tuberculoma, coccidioidoma
         b. Cryptococcosis, blastomycosis, actinomycosis
      2. Unidentified granulomas
   B. Common
      1. Lung abscess before evacuation into a bronchus
      2. Slowly resolving circumscribed pneumonia
      3. Lipoid pneumonia
      4. Hamartoma
   C. Less common
      1. Bronchogenic cyst
      2. Pulmonary infarct
      3. Bronchial adenoma
      4. A-V fistula
      5. Enlarged pulmonary artery
      6. Infected, fluid-filled bulla
      7. Rheumatoid nodule

*Modified from: Oches RN. In Fishman AP, editor: *Pulmonary diseases and disorders*, ed 2, vol 3. New York, 1988, McGraw-Hill, p. 2019.
†Source: Rohwedder JJ. In Guenter CA, Welch MH, editors: *Pulmonary Medicine*, ed 2. Philadelphia, 1982, J. B. Lippincott, p. 843.

VII-24 DIFFERENTIAL DIAGNOSIS OF TUMORS METASTATIC TO THE LUNGS

I. Parenchymal nodules
 A. Solitary carcinoma
  1. Large bowel
  2. Breast
  3. Kidney
  4. Female genital tract
  5. Skin
 B. Solitary sarcoma
  1. Osteogenic
 C. Multiple nodules
  1. Any carcinoma
  2. Any sarcoma
II. Endobronchial metastases
 A. Carcinoma
  1. Kidney
  2. Large bowel
 B. Fibrosarcoma
 C. Malignant melanoma
III. Lymphangitic metastases (carcinomas)
 A. Lung
 B. Stomach
 C. Breast
 D. Large bowel
 E. Pancreas

Modified from: Ochs R. In Fishman AP, editor: *Pulmonary diseases and disorders*, ed 2, vol 3. New York, 1988, McGraw-Hill, p. 2022.

VII-25 DIFFERENTIAL DIAGNOSIS OF A MEDIASTINAL MASS

I. Situated predominantly in the anterior compartment
   A. Thymoma
   B. Germ cell neoplasm
      1. Teratoma
      2. Seminoma
      3. Primary choriocarcinoma
      4. Endodermal sinus tumor
   C. Thyroid masses
   D. Parathyroid masses
   E. Mesenchymal neoplasms
      1. Lipoma
      2. Fibroma
      3. Hemangioma
      4. Lymphangioma
      5. Angiosarcoma
II. Situated predominantly in the middle compartment
   A. Lymph node enlargement caused by lymphoma or leukemia
   B. Lymph node enlargement caused by metastatic carcinoma
   C. Lymph node enlargement caused by infections
      1. Fungal
      2. Tuberculosis
      3. Mononucleosis
   D. Lymph node enlargement caused by granulomatous disease
   E. Primary tracheal neoplasms
   F. Bronchogenic cyst
   G. Masses situated in the anterior cardiophrenic angle
   H. Dilatation of the main pulmonary artery
   I. Dilatation of the major mediastinal veins
   J. Dilatation of the aorta or its branches
III. Situated predominantly in the posterior compartment
   A. Neurogenic neoplasms
   B. Meningocele
   C. Neurenteric cysts
   D. Gastroenteric cysts
   E. Thoracic duct cysts
   F. Primary lesions of the esophagus
      1. Neoplasm
      2. Diverticula
      3. Megaesophagus
      4. Hiatal hernia
   G. Hernia through the foramen of Bochdalek

VII-25 DIFFERENTIAL DIAGNOSIS OF A MEDIASTINAL MASS (CONTINUED)

H. Diseases of the thoracic spine
   1. Neoplasms
   2. Infectious spondylitis
   3. Fracture with hematoma
I. Extramedullary hematopoiesis

Adapted from: Fraser RG, Para JA. In Fraser RG, Pare JAP, Fraser RS, Genereau GP, editors: *Diagnosis of Diseases of the Chest* ed 3, vol IV. 1991, p. 2794.

VII-26 PULMONARY MANIFESTATIONS OF THE COLLAGEN-VASCULAR DISEASES

Pulmonary manifestations	Rheumatoid arthritis	Systemic sclerosis	Polymyositis and dermatomyositis	Systemic lupus erythematosus
Pleural				
Thickening	++	+	0	++
Effusion	++	0	0	+++
Parenchymal				
Acute pneumonia	0	0	0	+
Diffuse interstitial fibrosis	++*	+++	++*	+
Nodules	++	0	0	0
Primary pulmonary vasculopathy	0	++	0	+
Aspiration	0	++	+++	0
Ventilatory insufficiency	0	+	++	+

*A rapidly progressing variant may occur.

Note: O = Absent or rare. + = uncommon; ++ = recognized manifestation; +++ = important feature of disease.

From: Dickey B Myers A. In Fishman AP, editor: *Pulmonary diseases and disorders*, ed 2, vol 1. New York, 1988, McGraw-Hill, p. 646.

VII-27 PULMONARY-RENAL SYNDROMES

I. Goodpasture's syndrome (antiglomerular membrane disease)
II. Vasculitides
III. Polyarteritis nodosa
IV. Churg-Strauss
V. Hypersensitivity angiitis (Zeek's syndrome, Schönlein-Henoch purpura, essential mixed cryoglobulinemia, "collagen diseases", malignancy, liver disease)
VI. Wegener's granulomatosis
VII. Lymphomatoid granulomatosis
VIII. Behçet's syndrome
IX. Systemic lupus erythematosus
X. Progressive systemic sclerosis (scleroderma)
XI. Mixed connective tissue disease

Modified from: Matthay RA. *Yale J Biol Med* 53:497,1980

VII-28 IMITATORS OF PULMONARY-RENAL SYNDROMES

I. Infections
  A. Bacterial endocarditis with pneumonitis and GN
  B. Strep pneumonia with GN
  C. Staph pneumonia/abscess with GN
  D. Tuberculosis
  E. Leprosy
  F. Leptospirosis
  G. Legionnaires
  H. Hepatitis B
II. Sarcoid
III. CHF
IV. ARDS & ARF
V. Drugs
VI. Renal vein thrombosis with pulmonary embolism
VII. Plasma cell dyscrasia
VIII. Amyloid
IX. Fabry's disease

Modified from: Matthay RA. *Yale J Biol Med* 53:497,1980.

VII-29 DIFFERENTIAL DIAGNOSIS OF FEVER AND PULMONARY INFILTRATES IN RENAL TRANSPLANTS*

CXR	Acute (< 24 hrs)	Chronic (days-weeks)
focal/multifocal	bacterial thromboembolic pulmonary edema	fungal nocardial TB
diffuse	pulmonary edema	viral pneumocystis
nodular	(bacterial, pulmonary edema)	(fungal) nocardial
peribronchovascular	pulmonary edema (bacterial)	viral pneumocystis
consolidation	bacterial thromboembolic (pulmonary edema)	fungal nocardial (viral)

(...) represents atypical manifestations
*Pulmonary embolic disease and edema account for 27%
*96% mortality for patients developing a secondary infection

Modified from: Roasey PG, et al. *Medicine* 59:206, 1980.

VII-30 DRUGS IMPLICATED IN THE ETIOLOGY OF PULMONARY PARENCHYMAL INJURY

Cytotoxic   Noncytoxic

I. Antibiotics
   A. Bleomycin
   B. Mitomycin
   C. Neocarzinostatin
II. Alkylating agents
   A. Busulfan
   B. Cyclophosphamide
   C. Chlorambucil
   D. Melphalan
III. Nitrosoureas
   A. Carmustine (BCR/U)
   B. Lomostine (CCR/U)
   C. Chlorozotocin
IV. Antimetabolites
   A. Methotrexate
   B. Azathioprine
   C. Mercaptopurine
   D. Cytosine arabinoside
V. Miscellaneous
   A. Procarbazine
   B. Vinblastine

I. Antibacterial
   A. Nitrofurantoin
   B. Amphotericin
   C. Sulfasalazine
II. Analgesics
   A. Aspirin
III. Opiates
   A. Heroin
   B. Propoxyphene
   C. Methadone
IV. Sedatives
   A. Ethchlorvynol
   B. Chlordiazepoxide
V. Anticonvulsants
   A. Diphenylhydantoin
   B. Carbamazepine
VI. Diuretics
   A. Hydrochlorothiazide
VII. Major Tranquilizers
   A. Haloperidol
   B. Fluphenazine
VIII. Antiarrhythmics
   A. Amiodarone
   B. Lidocaine
   C. Tocainide
IX. Miscellaneous
   A. Gold salts
   B. Penicillamine
   C. Colchicine

Modified from: Cooper JAD, et al. *Am Rev Respir Dis* 133:322, 1986.

VII-31 MULTI-ORGAN SYSTEM FAILURE:[†] MODIFIED APACHE II CRITERIA

I. Cardiovascular failure
   A. Heart rate $\leq$ 54/min
   B. Mean arterial blood pressure < 49 mm Hg
      (systolic blood pressure $\leq$ 60 mm Hg)
   C. Ventricular tachycardia and/or fibrillation
   D. Serum pH $\leq$ 7.24 with pCO_2 of $\leq$ 49 mm Hg

II. Respiratory failure
   A. Respiratory rate $\leq$ 5/min or $\geq$ 49/min
   B. $pCO_2 \geq$ 50 mm Hg
   C. $AaDO_2 \geq$ 350 mm Hg
      ($AaDO_2 = 713 \, FIO_2 - pCO_2 - pO_2$)
   D. Ventilator or CPAP dependent 48 hours after appearance of
      another criterion

III. Renal failure*
   A. Urine output $\leq$ 479 ml/24 hours or $\leq$ 159 ml/8 hours
   B. Serum BUN $\geq$ 100 mg/100 ml
   C. Serum creatinine $\geq$ 3.5 mg/100 ml

IV. Hematologic failure
   A. WBC $\leq$ 1,000 cu mm
   B. Platelets $\leq$ 20,000 cu mm
   C. Hematocrit $\leq$ 20%

V. Neurologic failure
   A. Glasgow Coma Score $\leq$ 6 (in absence of sedation)

VI. Liver failure
   A. Bilirubin > 6 mg%
   B. PT > 4 sec over control

[†]Presence of any one or more of the criteria during a 24-hour period signifies
organ failure.
*Excluding patients on chronic dialysis prior to hospitalization.

Modified from: Knaus WA, Wagner DP. Multiple systems organ failure:
epidemiology: prognosis. *Crit Care Clin* 5(2):223, April 1989.

CHAPTER VIII
CLINICAL IMMUNOLOGY
AND RHEUMATOLOGY

VIII-1 DIAGNOSTIC CRITERIA FOR SYSTEMIC LUPUS ERYTHEMATOSUS

I. Malar rash
II. Discoid rash
III. Photosensitivity
IV. Oral or nasopharyngeal ulcers
V. Arthritis
VI. Serositis
   A. Pleuritis *or*
   B. Pericarditis
VII. Renal disorder
   A. Proteinuria > 0.5 grams/day *or*
   B. Cellular casts
VIII. Neurologic disorder
   A. Seizures *or*
   B. Psychosis
IX. Hematologic disorder, one of the following
   A. Hemolytic anemia
   B. Leukopenia
   C. Lymphopenia
   D. Thrombocytopenia
X. Immunologic disorder, one of the following
   A. Positive LE prep
   B. Antibody to DNA
   C. Antibody to SM
   D. False positive serologic test for syphilis
XI. Antinuclear antibody in abnormal titer

Four or more are required for the diagnosis of systemic lupus erythematosus.

Reference: Tan EM, et al. The 1982 revised criteria for the classification of systemic lupus erythematosus. *Arthritis Rheum* 25:1271-1277, 1982.

VIII-2 UNDERLYING CONDITIONS ASSOCIATED WITH RAYNAUD'S PHENOMENON

I. Connective tissue diseases
   A. Scleroderma
   B. Lupus erythematosus
   C. Dermatomyositis
   D. Rheumatoid arthritis
   E. Mixed connective tissue disease
   F. Sjögren's syndrome

II. Neurogenic disorders
   A. Thoracic outlet syndrome
   B. Carpal tunnel syndrome
   C. Reflex sympathetic dystrophy

III. Vaso-occlusive disease
   A. Arteriosclerosis obliterans
   B. Thromboangiitis obliterans
   C. Peripheral emboli

IV. Hematologic disorders
   A. Cryoglobulinemia
   B. Cold agglutinins
   C. Dysproteinemias

V. Drugs
   A. Ergot
   B. Heavy metal intoxications (lead and arsenic)
   C. Propranolol
   D. Sulfasalazine

VI. Occupational or environmental exposure
   A. Pneumatic hammer disease
   B. Disorders in typists and pianists
   C. Sequelae of blunt trauma or cold injury

VII. Miscellaneous
   A. Polycythemia vera
   B. Hypothyroidism
   C. Occult carcinoma
   D. Primary pulmonary hypertension
   E. Primary/idiopathic

Modified from: Creager MA, Pzau, VJ. In Braunwald E, Isselbacher KJ, Petersdorf RG, Wilson JD, Martin J, Fauci AS, Root RK, editors: *Harrison's principles of internal medicine*, ed 12. New York, 1991, McGraw-Hill, p. 1022.

VIII-3 POLYMYALGIA RHEUMATICA

I. Diagnostic Criteria
   A. Musculoskeletal pain in neck, shoulders, and pelvic girdle for at least one month.
   B. Patients usually at least 60 years of age
   C. Elevated ESR (usually greater than 50)
   D. Frequently present
      1. Anemia
      2. Headache
      3. Morning stiffness > 1 hour
      4. Depression and/or weight loss
II. Differential Diagnosis
   A. Connective tissue disorders
      1. Rheumatoid arthritis
      2. Polymyositis
      3. Vasculitis
      4. Lupus erythematosus
   B. Neoplastic disorders
      1. Multiple myeloma
      2. Occult tumors
   C. Infections
      1. Post viral syndromes (esp. influenza)
      2. Occult infection
   D. Miscellaneous
      1. Degenerative joint disease
      2. Fibromyalgia

VIII-4 CRITERIA FOR DIAGNOSIS OF STEVENS-JOHNSON SYNDROME

I. Major Criteria
   A. Skin lesions
   B. Erythema multiforme exudativum
   C. Stomatitis (ulcerative)
   D. Genital or anal ulcers
II. Minor Criteria
   A. Pneumonitis — preceding or coexistent
   B. History of upper respiratory or genitourinary infection treated with sulfonamides or antibiotics
   C. Arthralgias
   D. Conjunctivitis
   E. History of ingestion of wide variety of drugs, both prescription and nonprescripton

Adapted from: Ehrlich G. In McCarty DJ, editor: *Arthritis and allied conditions.* Philadelphia, 1985, Lea & Febiger, p. 896.

VIII-5 DIAGNOSIS OF BEHÇET'S SYNDROME

I. Major criteria:
   A. Mouth (aphthous) ulcers
   B. Iritis (with hypopyon)
   C. Genital ulcers
   D. Skin lesions
      1. Pyoderma
      2. Nodose lesions
II. Minor criteria:
   A. Arthritis
      1. Of major joints
      2. Arthralgias
   B. Vascular disease
      1. Migratory superficial phlebitis
      2. Major vessel thrombosis
      3. Aneurysms
      4. Peripheral gangrene
      5. Retinal and vitreous hemorrhage, papilledema
   C. Central nervous system disease
      1. Brain stem syndrome
      2. Meningomyelitis
      3. Confusional states
   D. Gastrointestinal disease
      1. Malabsorption
      2. Colonic ulcers
      3. Dilated intestinal loops
   E. Epididymitis
   F. Hemorrhagic pneumonitis
   G. Glomerulonephritis

Adapted from: Ehrlich G. In McCarty DJ, editor: *Arthritis and allied conditions*, ed 11. Philadelphia, 1989, Lea & Febiger, p. 999.

VIII-6 CRITERIA FOR THE DIAGNOSIS OF SCLERODERMA (PROGRESSIVE SYSTEMIC SCLEROSIS)

I. Single major criterion - proximal scleroderma*
II. Minor criteria
   A. Sclerodactyly
   B. Digital pitting of finger tips
   C. Bibasilar pulmonary fibrosis

*A term indicating bilateral and symmetric sclerodermatous changes in any area proximal to the metacarpal or metatarsal phalangeal joints. The diagnosis of definite scleroderma can be made with 1 major or 2 or more minor criteria. Reference: Masi AT, et al. *Arthritis Rheum* 23:581, 1980.

VIII-7 DIAGNOSTIC CRITERIA FOR INFLAMMATORY MYOPATHIES

Criterion	Polymyositis		Dermatomyositis		Inclusion-body myositis
	Definite	Probable*	Definite	Mild or early	Definite
I. Muscle strength	Myopathic muscle weakness†	Myopathic muscle weakness†	Myopathic muscle weakness†	Seemingly normal strength‡ of distal muscles†	Myopathic muscle weakness with early involvement
II. Electro-myo-graphic findings	Myopathic	Myopathic	Myopathic or nonspecific	Myopathic potentials	Myopathic with mixed
III. Muscle enzymes	Elevated (up to 50-fold)	Elevated (up to 50-fold) or normal	Elevated (up to 50-fold) or normal	Elevated (up to 10-fold) or normal	Elevated (up to 10-fold) or normal
IV. Muscle biopsy findings	Diagnostic for this type of inflammatory myopathy	Nonspecific myopathy without signs of primary inflammation	Diagnostic	Nonspecific or diagnostic	Diagnostic
V. Rash or calcinosis	Absent	Absent	Present	Present	Absent

VIII-7 DIAGNOSTIC CRITERIA FOR INFLAMMATORY MYOPATHIES (CONTINUED)

*An adequate trial of prednisone or other immunosuppressive drugs is warranted in probable cases. If, in retrospect, the disease is unresponsive to therapy, another muscle biopsy should be considered to exclude other diseases or possible evolution to inclusion body myositis.

†Myopathic muscle weakness, affecting proximal muscles more than distal ones and sparing eye and facial muscles, is characterized by a subacute onset (weeks to months) and rapid progression in patients who have no family history of neuromuscular disease, no endocrinopathy, no exposure to myotoxic drugs or toxins, and no biochemical muscle disease (excluded on the basis of muscle-biopsy findings).

‡Although strength is seemingly normal, patients often have new onset of easy fatigue, myalgia, and reduced endurance. Careful muscle testing may reveal mild muscle weakness.

From: Dalakas MC. *New Engl J Med* 325(21):1490, 1991.

VIII-8 REVISED CRITERIA FOR CLASSIFICATION OF RHEUMATOID ARTHRITIS (TRADITIONAL FORMAT)

Criterion	Definition
I. Morning stiffness	Morning stiffness in and around the joints, lasting at least 1 hour before maximal improvement.
II. Arthritis of 3 or more joint areas	At least 3 joint areas simultaneously have had soft tissue swelling or fluid (not bony overgrowth alone) observed by a physician. The 14 possible areas are right or left PIP, MCP, wrist, elbow, knee, ankle, and MTP joints.
III. Arthritis of hand joints	At least 1 area swollen (as defined above) in a wrist, MCP, or PIP joint.
IV. Symmetric arthritis	Simultaneous involvement of the same joint areas (as defined in 2) on both sides of the body.
V. Rheumatoid nodules	Subcutaneous nodules, over bony prominences, or extensor surfaces, or in juxtaarticular regions, observed by a physician.
VI. Serum rheumatoid factor	Demonstration of abnormal amounts of serum rheumatoid factor by any method for which the result has been positive in < 5% of normal control subjects
VII. Radiographic changes	Radiographic changes typical of rheumatoid arthritis on posteroanterior hand and wrist radiographs, which must include erosions or unequivocal bony decalcification localized in or most markedly adjacent to the involved joints (osteoarthritis changes alone do not qualify)

*For classification purposes, a patient shall be said to have rheumatoid arthritis if he/she has satisfied at least 4 of these 7 criteria. Criteria 1 through 4 must have been present for at least 6 weeks. Patients with 2 clinical diagnoses are not excluded. Designation as classic, definite, or probable rheumatoid arthritis is *not* to be made.

Joints: PIP = proximal interphalangeal; MCP = metacarpophalangeal; MTP = metatarsophalangeal.

From: Arnett FC, Edworthy SM, Bloch DA, et al. *Arthritis Rheum* 31: 315-324, March 1988.

VIII-9 CLINICAL FEATURES SUGGESTING REITER'S SYNDROME

   I. History of diarrhea or extramarital sexual intercourse prior to attack
   II. Fever
   III. Arthritis, usually pauciarticular
   IV. Urethritis, possibly complicated by cystitis, prostatic abscess or hydronephrosis
   V. Conjunctivitis, possibly complicated by keratitis, iritis, retinitis or optic neuritis
   VI. Skin lesions
      A. Keratoderma blennorhagicum
      B. Circinate balanitis
      C. Superficial ulcerations on tongue and buccal mucosa
   VII. Possible ECG changes, infrequently pericarditis

Yu, D.T. and Hoffman RW. In Schumacher HR Jr, editor: *Primer on the rheumatic diseases*, ed 9. Atlanta, 1988, Arthritis Foundation, p. 147-148.

VIII-10 DIAGNOSTIC* CRITERIA OF ANKYLOSING SPONDYLITIS

   I. Clinical Criteria
      A. Low back pain of over 3 months duration, unrelieved by rest, improved with exercise
      B. Limited chest expansion
      C. Limited motion of the lumbar spine
      D. Past or present evidence of iritis.
   II. Radiological Criteria
      A. Bilateral sacroiliitis grade 2-4
      B. Unilateral sacroiliitis grade 3-4

*Definite ankylosing spondylitis if either radiological criterion present with one clinical criterion.

Adapted from: Ball GV. In McCarty DJ, editor. *Arthritis and allied conditions*, ed 11. Philadelphia, 1989, Lea & Febiger, p. 935.

VIII-11 CRITERIA FOR DIAGNOSIS OF GOUTY ARTHRITIS

A patient with six or more variable positives would be classified as having gout.

    I. Monoarticular arthritis
   II. Occurrence of more than one attack
  III. Maximal inflammation developing within one day
   IV. Redness over joints
    V. Pain or swelling in the first metatarsophalangeal joint
   VI. Unilateral involvement of (5)
  VII. Unilateral involvement of a tarsal joint
 VIII. Tophus—either proved or suspected to contain MSU crystals
   IX. Serum uric acid > normal for that particular lab
    X. X-ray demonstrated asymmetric joint swelling
   XI. Subcortical cysts without erosions on x-ray
  XII. Monosodium urate crystals in joint fluid
 XIII. Joint fluid negative for organisms

Synovial fluid MSU cyrstals of proved tophus are universally accepted as the ultimate diagnosis for gout.

Reference: Schumacher HR, editor. *Primer on rheumatic diseases*, ed 9. Atlanta, 1988, Arthritis Foundation, p. 320.

VIII-12 PROVISIONAL CRITERIA FOR DIAGNOSIS OF PSORIATIC ARTHRITIS*

   I. Mandatory
      Clinically apparent psoriasis (skin or nails) in association with pain and soft tissue swelling and/or limitation of motion in at least one joint, observed by a physician for six weeks or longer
  II. Supportive
      A. Pain and soft tissue swelling and/or limitation of motion in one or more other joints, observed by a physician.
      B. Presence of an inflammatory arthritis in distal interphalangeal joint
      C. Specific exclusions—Heberden's or Bouchard's nodes
      D. Presence of "sausage" fingers or toes
      E. An asymmetric distribution of the arthritis in the hands and feet
      F. Absence of subcutaneous nodules
      G. A negative test for rheumatoid factor in the serum
      H. An inflammatory synovial fluid with a normal or increased C3 or C4 level, and an absence of: (a) infection, including AFB, (b) crystals of monosodium urate or calcium pyrophosphate

VIII-12 PROVISIONAL CRITERIA FOR DIAGNOSIS OF PSORIATIC ARTHRITIS* (CONTINUED)

I. A synovial biopsy showing synovial lining hypertrophy with a predominantly mononuclear cell infiltration, and an absence of: (a) granuloma formation, (b) tumor

J. Peripheral radiographs showing an erosive arthritis of small joints with a relative lack of osteoporosis. Specific exclusion - erosive osteoarthritis

*Definite psoriatic arthritis - mandatory plus six supportive criteria. Probable psoriatic arthritis - mandatory plus four supportive criteria. Possible psoriatic arthritis - mandatory plus two supportive criteria.

Adapted from: Bennett, R. In *Arthritis and Allied Conditions*, McCarty, D.J. (ed.), 11th Edition, Lea & Febiger, Philadelphia, 1989, p. 956.

VIII-13 DIFFERENTIAL DIAGNOSIS OF INFLAMMATORY MONOARTHRITIS

I. Crystal induced
   A. Gout
   B. Pseudogout
   C. Calcific tendinitis
II. Palindromic rheumatism
III. Infectious arthritis
   A. Septic
   B. Tubercular
   C. Fungal
   D. Viral
IV. Other
   A. Tendinitis
   B. Bursitis
   C. Juvenile rheumatoid arthritis

Modified from: McCarty, D. In McCarty DJ, editor. *Arthritis and allied conditions*, ed 11. Philadelphia, 1989, Lea & Febiger, p. 65.

VIII-14 DIAGNOSTIC FEATURES OF SARCOIDOSIS

I. Sarcoidosis
   A. Noncaseating granulomas on biopsy. Must exclude other causes of granulomas
   B. Hilar and right paratracheal adenopathy in 90%
   C. Skin lesions, uveitis, or involvement of almost any tissue
   D. Onset most often in third and fourth decades, but cases reported at all ages.
   E. Impaired delayed hypersensitivity in 85%
   F. Frequent hyperglobulinemia
   G. Increased angiotensin-converting enzyme levels in about 80%.
   H. Hypercalciuria in most; hypercalcemia in some
II. Sarcoid arthropathy
   Acute Sarcoidosis (Lofgren's Syndrome, hilar adenopathy, fever, erythema nodosum)
   A. Often periarticular and very tender, warm swelling.
   B. Ankles and knees almost invariably involved.
   C. May be initial manifestation
   D. Joint motion may be normal
   E. Synovial effusions infrequent and usually mildly inflammatory when present
   F. Usually nonspecific mild synovitis on synovial biopsy
   G. Self-limited in weeks to 4 months
III. Chronic sarcoidosis
   A. May be acute and evanescent, recurrent or chronic
   B. Noncaseating granulomas more commonly demonstrable in synovium
   C. Usually nondestructive despite chronic or recurrent disease

Adapted from: Schumacher H. In McCarty DJ, editor. *Arthritis and allied conditions*, ed 11. Philadelphia, 1989, Lea & Febiger, pp. 1296-1298.

VIII-15 DIFFERENTIAL DIAGNOSIS OF POSITIVE BLOOD TEST FOR RHEUMATOID FACTOR

I. Rheumatologic Disease
   A. Rheumatoid arthritis
   B. Juvenile rheumatoid arthritis
   C. Systemic lupus erythematosus
   D. Mixed connective tissue disease
   E. Behçet's syndrome
   F. Sjögren's syndrome
II. Infectious Disease
   A. Bacterial (especially endocarditis)
   B. Syphilis
   C. Viral hepatitis
   D. Parasitic infections
   E. Granulomatous disease
   F. Mononucleosis
   G. AIDS
III. Pulmonary Disease
   A. Bronchitis or asthma
   B. Coal miner's disease
   C. Asbestosis
   D. Idiopathic pulmonary fibrosis
   E. Sarcoidosis
IV. Other Diseases
   A. Cirrhosis
   B. Myocardial infarction
   C. Neoplasms
   D. Essential mixed cryoglobulinemia
V. Healthy Persons — Increases with age

Modified from: Coffey R, et al. *Postgraduate Medicine* 70:164, 1981.

VIII-16 CRYOGLOBULINEMIA

I. Essential or idiopathic
II. Secondary to or associated with
   A. Hemopoietic disorders
      1. Multiple myeloma
      2. Waldenström's macroglobulinemia
      3. Lymphatic leukemia, lymphosarcoma
      4. Polycythemia vera
      5. Sickle cell anemia
   B. Connective tissue disorders
      1. Systemic lupus erythematosus
      2. Syndrome of arthralgia, purpura, nephritis, and weakness
      3. Rheumatoid arthritis
      4. Ankylosing spondylitis
      5. Polyarteritis nodosa
      6. Sjögren's syndrome
      7. Thyroiditis
      8. Lymphoepithelial tumors of parotid gland
      9. Acute poststreptococcal glomerulonephritis
   C. Chronic infections
      1. Subacute bacterial endocarditis
      2. Visceral leishmaniasis (kala-azar)
      3. Syphilis
      4. Toxoplasmosis
      5. Leprosy
      6. Malaria
      7. Schistosomiasis
      8. Lyme's disease
      9. HIV
   D. Others
      1. Chronic liver disease (cirrhosis, cholecystitis, chronic hepatitis, gallbladder neoplasm)
      2. Skin disorders (porphyria cutanea tarda, pemphigus, erythrodermia)
      3. Acute myocardial infarction
      4. Infectious mononucleosis
      5. Ulcerative colitis
      6. Sarcoidosis
      7. Cytomegalovirus infection

Modified from: Meyers AR. In Schumacher HR Jr, editor: *Primer on rheumatic diseases, ed 9.* Atlanta, 1988, Arthritis Foundation, p. 132.

VIII-17 CLASSIFICATION OF THE VASCULITIC SYNDROMES

I. Systemic necrotizing vasculitis
   A. Classic polyarteritis nodosa
   B. Allergic angiitis and granulomatosis of Churg-Strauss
   C. Polyangiitis overlap syndrome
II. Hypersensitivity vasculitis
   A. Exogenous stimuli proved or suspected
      1. Schölein-Henoch purpura
      2. Serum sickness and serum sickness-like reactions
      3. Other drug-induced vasculitides
      4. Vasculitis associated with infectious diseases
   B. Endogenous antigens likely involved
      1. Vasculitis associated with neoplasms
      2. Vasculitis associated with connective tissue diseases
      3. Vasculitis associated with other underlying diseases
      4. Vasculitis associated with congenital deficiencies of the complement system
III. Wegener's granulomatosis
IV. Giant cell arteritis
   A. Temporal arteritis
   B. Takayasu's arteritis
V. Other vasculitis syndromes
   A. Mucocutaneous lymph node syndrome (Kawasaki's disease)
   B. Isolated central nervous system vasculitis
   C. Thromboangiitis obliterans (Buerger's disease)
   D. Miscellaneous vasculitides

From: Fauci AS. In *Harrison's principles of internal medicine*, 12th Edition, McGraw-Hill, New York, 1991, p. 1457.

VIII-18 AUTOANTIBODIES IN RHEUMATIC DISEASES: DISEASE ASSOCIATIONS AND MOLECULAR IDENTIFICATION

Antibody to:	Disease association (percent prevalence)
I. Native double-stranded DNA (dsDNA)	SLE (> 50%)*
II. Histones	SLE(70%)
	Drug-induced SLE (> 95%)
III. Sm (Smith)	SLE (30%)*
IV. Nuclear RNP	SLE (30%)
V. Ro/SSA (ribonuclear protein)	Mixed connective tissue disease (> 95%)
	SLE (35%)
	Sjögren's syndrome (60%)
	Complete congenital heart block (> 85%)
	Subacute cutaneous LE (85%)
VI. La/SSB	SLE (15%)
	Sjögren's syndrome (40%)
	Complete congenital heart block
VII. Jo_1 (Histidyl-tRNA Synthetase)	Dermatomyositis/Polymyositis (25%)*
VIII. Scl_{70}	Scleroderma (20%)*
IX. Centromere kinetochore	CREST (70% to 90%)
	Diffuse scleroderma (10% to 20%)
X. Antineutrophil cytoplasmic antibody (ANCA)	Wegener granulomatosis (> 90%)
	Limited Wegener (60%)
	Other vasculitides (low)
XI. Phospholipid (cardiolipid)	SLE (30% to 40%)
	Unexplained fetal death (10% to 15%), vascular occlusion

*Disease-specific

From: *Medical knowledge self-assessment program (IX)*, Part B, Book 6. American College of Physicians, 1991, p. 571.

VIII-19 PUTATIVE ASSOCIATIONS OF CPPD CRYSTAL DEPOSITION

I. Group A (true association — high probability)
   A. Hyperparathyroidism
   B. Hemochromatosis
   C. Hemosiderosis
   D. Hypophosphatasia
   E. Hypomagnesemia
   F. Hypothyroidism
   G. Gout
   H. Neuropathic joints
   I. Aging
   J. Amyloidosis
   K. Trauma/Surgery
   L. Familial hypocalciuric hypercalcemia
II. Group B (true association — modest probability)
   A. Hyperthyroidism
   B. Renal stone
   C. Ankylosing hyperostosis
   D. Ochronosis
   E. Wilson's disease
   F. Hemophilia arthritis
III. Group C (true association — unlikely)
   A. Diabetes mellitus
   B. Hypertension
   C. Mild azotemia
   D. Hyperuricemia
   E. Gynecomastia
   F. Inflammatory bowel disease
   G. Rheumatoid arthritis
   H. Paget's disease of bone
   I. Acromegaly

(CPPD = calcium pyrophosphate dihydrate.)

Modified from: Ryan LM, McCarty DJ. In McCarty DJ, editor. *Arthritis and allied conditions*, ed 11. Philadelphia, 1989, Lea & Febiger, p. 1730.

VIII-20 SYNOVIAL FLUID CHARACTERISTICS

	Normal	Group I Noninflammatory	Group II Inflammatory	Group III Septic
Gross appearance	Transparent, clear	Transparent, yellow	Opaque or translucent, yellow	Opaque, yellow to green
Viscosity	High	High	Low	Variable
White cells/mm^3	< 200	< 200	5,000–75,000	> 50,000, often > 100,000
Polymorphonuclear leukocytes	< 25%	< 25%	> 50%	> 75%
Culture	Negative	Negative	Negative	Often positive
Glucose (mg/dl)	Nearly equal to blood	Nearly equal to blood	> 25, lower than blood	> 50, lower than blood
Associated conditions		Degenerative joint disease Trauma Neuropathic arthropathy	Rheumatoid arthritis Connective tissue diseases (SLE, PSS, DM/PM)	Bacterial infections Compromised immunity (disease or medication related)

VIII-20 SYNOVIAL FLUID CHARACTERISTICS (CONTINUED)

Normal	Group I Noninflammatory	Group II Inflammatory	Group III Septic
	Hypertrophic osteoarthropathy Pigmented villonodular synovitis SLE Acute rheumatic fever	Ankylosing spondylitis Other seronegative spondyloarthropathies (psoriatic arthritis, Reiter's syndrome, arthritis of chronic inflammatory bowel disease)	Other joint disease
	Erythema nodosum	Crystal-induced synovitis (gout or pseudogout) Acute rheumatic fever	

Adapted from: McCarty DJ. In McCarty DJ, editor. Arthritis and allied conditions, ed 11. Philadelphia, 1989, Lea & Febiger, p. 71, 74.

VIII-21 THE AMERICAN COLLEGE OF RHEUMATOLOGY 1990 CRITERIA FOR THE CLASSIFICATION OF FIBROMYALGIA*

I. History of widespread pain
   A. Definition. Pain is considered widespread when all of the following are present: pain in the left side of the body, pain in the right side of the body, pain above the waist, and pain below the waist. In addition, axial skeletal pain (cervical spine or anterior chest or thoracic spine or low back) must be present. In this definition, shoulder and buttock pain is considered as pain for each involved side. "Low back" pain is considered lower segment pain.

II. Pain in 11 of 18 tender point sites on digital palpation.
   A. Definition. Pain, on digital palpation, must be present in at least 11 of the following 18 tender point sites:
      1. Occiput: Bilateral, at the suboccipital muscle insertions.
      2. Low cervical: Bilateral, at the anterior aspects of the intertransverse spaces at C5-C7.
      3. Trapezius: Bilateral, at the midpoint of the upper border.
      4. Supraspinatus: Bilateral, at origins, above the scapula spine near the medial border.
      5. Second rib: Bilateral, at the second costochondral junctions, just lateral to the junctions on upper surfaces.
      6. Lateral epicondyle: Bilateral, 2 cm distal to the epicondyles.
      7. Gluteal: Bilateral, in upper outer quadrants of buttocks in anterior fold of muscle.
      8. Greater trochanter: Bilateral, posterior to the trochanteric prominence.
      9. Knee: Bilateral, at the medial fat pad proximal to the joint line.

Digital palpation should be performed with an approximate force of 4 kg.

For a tender point to be considered "positive" the subject must state that the palpation was painful. "Tender" is not to be considered "painful."

*For classification purposes, patients will be said to have fibromyalgia if both criteria are satisfied. Widespread pain must have been present for at least 3 months. The presence of a second clinical disorder does not exclude the diagnosis of fibromyalgia.

Reference: Wolfe F, et al. *Arthritis and Rheumatism*, 33(2):171, 1990.

CHAPTER IX
NEUROLOGY

IX-1 CLASSIFICATION OF COMA AND DIFFERENTIAL DIAGNOSIS

I. Diseases that cause no focal or lateralizing neurologic signs or alteration of the cellular content of the CSF. Usually brain stem functions and CT are normal
   A. Intoxications: Alcohol, barbiturates, opiates, etc.
   B. Metabolic disturbances: Anoxia, diabetic acidosis, uremia, hepatic coma, hypoglycemia, Addisonian crisis, hyperosmolar non-ketotic coma, hypercapnia, hypernatremia, myxedema coma
   C. Severe systemic infections: Pneumonia, typhoid fever, malaria, septicemia, Waterhouse-Friderichsen syndrome
   D. Circulatory collapse from any cause, and cardiac decompensation in the aged
   E. Epilepsy: Postictal states
   F. Hypertensive encephalopathy and eclampsia
   G. Hyperthermia or hypothermia
   H. Concussion

II. Diseases that cause meningeal irritation with blood or an excess of white cells in the CSF, usually without focal or lateralizing cerebral or brain stem signs. The CT scan may be normal or abnormal.
   A. Subarachnoid hemorrhage from ruptured aneurysm, AV malformation, occasionally trauma
   B. Acute bacterial meningitis
   C. Some forms of viral encephalitis

III. Diseases that cause focal brain stem or lateralizing cerebral signs, with or without changes in the CSF. CT scan is usually abnormal.
   A. Brain hemorrhage
   B. Cerebral infarction due to thrombosis or embolism
   C. Brain abscess, subdural empyema
   D. Epidural and subdural hemorrhage and brain contusion
   E. Brain tumor
   F. Miscellaneous: e.g., thrombophlebitis, some forms of viral encephalitis, focal embolic encephalomalacia due to bacterial endocarditis, acute hemorrhagic leukoencephalitis, disseminated (postinfectious) encephalomyelitis

Modified from: Adams R, Victor M. *Principles of neurology*, ed 4. New York, 1989, McGraw-Hill, p. 285.

IX-2 DIFFERENTIAL DIAGNOSIS OF MENINGITIS

I. Bacterial Meningitis
- A. Neisseria meningitidis
- B. Hemophilus influenzae
- C. Streptococcus pneumoniae
- D. Staphylococcus aureus and epidermidis
- E. Gram negatives
  1. Escherichia coli
  2. Klebsiella, Proteus, Pseudomonas
- F. Mycobacteria
- G. Leptospirosis
- H. Rare
  1. Listeria monocytogenes
  2. Mima-Herellea

II. Viral (Aseptic) Meningitis
- A. Enteroviruses
  1. Coxsackie viruses
  2. Echo viruses
- B. Herpes simplex
  1. Meningitis or meningoencephalitis
- C. Cytomegalovirus
- D. Epstein-Barr virus
- E. Measles
- F. Mumps
- G. Influenza
- H. Varicella zoster
- I. Rubella
- J. Adenovirus

III. Non-viral Agents Which May Cause Encephalitis-Aseptic Meningitis Syndromes
- A. Rickettsial
  1. Rocky Mountain Spotted Fever
  2. Q fever
- B. Chlamydia and mycoplasma
  1. Mycoplasma pneumoniae
  2. Psittacosis
- C. Mollaret recurrent meningitis
- D. Vogt-Koyanagi Harada syndrome

IX-3 DIFFERENTIAL DIAGNOSIS OF PERIPHERAL NEUROPATHIES

   I. Drugs (Nitrofurantoin, INH, pyridoxine in excess, vincristine, etc.)
   II. Alcohol
   III. Nutritional (pernicious anemia, thiamine, B_6)
   IV. Guillain-Barré syndrome
   V. Toxins (heavy metals — arsenic, lead, etc.)
   VI. Hereditary
   VII. Endocrine (diabetes mellitus, hypothyroidism)
   VIII. Renal failure
   IX. Amyloidosis
   X. Porphyria
   XI. Infections (syphilis, mononucleosis, diphtheria, leprosy)
   XII. Systemic disorders (rheumatoid arthritis, SLE, vasculitis, sarcoidosis)
   XII. Tumors

Mnemonic to remember the classification order: DANG THERAPIST

Modified from: Griffin JW. In Harvey AM, Johns R, McKusick V, Owens A, Ross R, editors: *The principles and practice of medicine*, ed 21. Norwalk, Conn., 1984, Appleton-Century-Crofts, p. 1315.

IX-4 CLASSIFICATION OF DEMENTIA

   I. Diseases in which dementia is associated with clinical and laboratory signs of other medical disease.
      A. Hypothyroidism
      B. Cushing syndrome
      C. Nutritional deficiency states such as pellagra, the Wernicke-Korsakoff syndrome, and subacute combined degeneration of spinal cord and brain (vitamin B_{12} deficiency)
      D. Chronic meningoencephalitis: general paresis, meningovascular syphilis, cryptococcosis
      E. Hepatolenticular degeneration, familial and acquired
      F. Chronic drug intoxication
   II. Diseases in which dementia is associated with other neurologic signs but not with other obvious medical disease
      A. Invariably associated with other neurologic signs
         1. Huntington chorea (choreoathetosis)
         2. Schilder disease and related demyelinative diseases (spastic weakness, pseudobulbar palsy, blindness, deafness)
         3. Amaurotic familial idiocy and other lipid-storage diseases (myoclonic seizures, blindness, spasticity, cerebellar ataxia)

IX-4 CLASSIFICATION OF DEMENTIA (CONTINUED)

      4. Myoclonic epilepsy (diffuse myoclonus, generalized seizures, cerebellar ataxia)
      5. Subacute spongiform encephalopathy or one type of Creutzfeldt-Jakob disease (myoclonic dementia)
      6. Cerebrocerebellar degeneration (cerebellar ataxia)
      7. Cerebral-basal ganglionic degenerations (apraxia-rigidity)
      8. Dementia with spastic paraplegia (spastic legs)
      9. Progressive supranuclear palsy
     10. Certain hereditary metabolic diseases

   B. Often associated with other neurologic signs
      1. Thrombotic or embolic cerebral infarction
      2. Brain tumor (primary or metastatic) or abscess
      3. Brain trauma, such as cerebral contusion, midbrain hemorrhage, chronic subdural hematoma
      4. Marchiafava-Bignami disease (often with apraxia and other frontal lobe signs)
      5. Communicating (normal-pressure) or obstructive hydrocephalus (usually with ataxia of gait)
      6. Progressive multifocal leukoencephalopathy

III. Diseases in which dementia is usually the only evidence of neurologic or medical disease
   A. Alzheimer disease
   B. Pick disease
   C. AIDS dementia
   D. Alcoholic dementia

Modified from: Adams R, Victor M. *Principles of neurology*, ed 4. New York, 1989, McGraw-Hill, p. 340.

IX-5 CLASSIFICATION OF DELIRIUM AND ACUTE CONFUSIONAL STATES

  I. Delirium
   A. In a medical or surgical illness (no focal or lateralizing neurologic sign; CSF usually clear)
      1. Typhoid fever
      2. Pneumonia
      3. Septicemia, particularly erysipelas and other streptococcal infections
      4. Rheumatic fever
      5. Thyrotoxicosis and ACTH intoxication (rare)
      6. Postoperative and postconcussive states
   B. In neurologic disease that causes focal or lateralizing signs or changes in the CSF

IX-5 CLASSIFICATION OF DELIRIUM AND ACUTE CONFUSIONAL STATES (CONTINUED)

1. Vascular, neoplastic, or other diseases, particularly those involving the temporal and parietal lobes and upper part of the brain stem
2. Cerebral contusion and laceration (traumatic delirium)
3. Acute purulent and tuberculous meningitis
4. Subarachnoid hemorrhage
5. Encephalitis due to viral causes (e.g., herpes simplex, infectious mononucleosis) and to unknown causes

C. The abstinence states, exogenous intoxications, and postconvulsive states; signs of other medical, surgical and neurologic illnesses absent or coincidental

1. Withdrawal of alcohol (delirium tremens), barbiturates, and nonbarbiturate sedative drugs, following chronic intoxication.
2. Drug intoxications: scopolamine, atropine, amphetamine, etc.
3. Postconvulsive delirium

II. Acute confusional states associated with psychomotor underactivity

A. Associated with a medical or surgical disease (no focal or lateralizing neurologic signs; CSF clear)

1. Metabolic disorders; hepatic stupor, uremia, hypoxia, hypercapnia, hypoglycemia, porphyria
2. Infective fevers, especially typhoid
3. Congestive heart failure
4. Postoperative, posttraumatic, and puerperal psychoses

B. Associated with drug intoxication (no focal or lateralizing signs; CSF clear): opiates, barbiturates and other sedatives, Artane, etc.

III. Associated with diseases of the nervous system (with focal or lateralizing neurologic signs and/or CSF changes)

A. Cerebral vascular disease, tumor, abscess
B. Subdural hematoma
C. Meningitis
D. Encephalitis

IV. Beclouded dementia, i.e., senile or other brain disease in combination with infective fevers, drug reactions, heart failure, or other medical or surgical diseases.

Modified from: Adams R, Victor M. *Principles of neurology*, ed 4. New York, 1989, McGraw-Hill, p. 329.

IX-6 SECONDARY CAUSES OF DEPRESSION

I. Neurologic diseases
   A. Neuronal degenerations — Alzheimer, Huntington, and Parkinson disease
   B. Focal CNS disease — strokes, brain tumors, and trauma, multiple sclerosis

II. Metabolic and endocrine diseases
   A. Corticosteroids, excess or deficiency
   B. Hypothyroidism, rarely thyrotoxicosis
   C. Cushing syndrome
   D. Addison disease
   E. Hyperparathyroidism
   F. Pernicious anemia
   G. Chronic renal failure/dialysis
   H. B-vitamin deficiencies

III. Myocardial infarction, open heart surgery, and other operations

IV. Infectious diseases
   A. Brucellosis
   B. Viral hepatitis, influenza, pneumonia
   C. Infectious mononucleosis

V. Cancer, particularly pancreatic

VI. Parturition

VII. Medications
   A. Analgesics and anti-inflammatory agents (other than steroids) — indomethacin, phenacetin, and phenylbutazone
   B. Amphetamines (when withdrawn)
   C. Antibiotics, particularly cycloserine, ethionamide, griseofulvin, isoniazid, nalidixic acid, and sulfonamides
   D. Antihypertensive drugs — clonidine, methyldopa, propranolol, reserpine
   E. Cardiac drugs — digitalis, procainamide
   F. Corticosteroids and ACTH
   G. Disulfiram
   H. L-Dopa
   I. Methysergide
   J. Oral contraceptives

Modified from: Adams R, Victor M. *Principles of neurology*, ed 4. New York, 1989, McGraw-Hill, p. 120.

IX-7 CAUSES OF HYPOGLYCORRHACHIA (DECREASED CEREBROSPINAL FLUID GLUCOSE)

I. Pyogenic meningitis
II. Tubercular meningitis
III. Fungal meningitis
IV. Sarcoidosis
V. Subarachnoid hemorrhage (recent)
VI. Meningeal carcinomatosis
VII. Occasional Causes
  A. Mumps meningoencephalitis
  B. Herpes encephalitis
  C. Zoster encephalitis

Modified from: Adams R, Victor M. *Principles of neurology*, ed 4. New York, 1989, McGraw-Hill, p. 14.

CHAPTER X
DERMATOLOGY

X-1 CONDITIONS ASSOCIATED WITH ERYTHEMA NODOSUM

I. Drugs Causing:
   A. Estrogens
   B. Oral contraceptives
   C. Sulfonamides
   D. Aminopyrine*
   E. Antimony compounds*
   F. Arsphenamine*
   G. Bromides*
   H. Immunizations*
   I. Iodides*
   J. Phenacetin*
   K. Salicylates*
   L. Vaccines*
II. Infections:
   A. Bacterial:
      1. Streptococcal infection
      2. Tuberculosis
      3. Yersinia (Pasteurella) infection (esp. Scandinavia), Y. enterocolitica and Y. pseudotuberculosis
      4. Brucellosis*
      5. Leptospirosis*
      6. Tularemia*
   B. Chlamydial
   C. Fungal:
      1. Coccidioidomycosis
      2. Histoplasmosis
      3. Dermatophytosis*
      4. North American blastomycosis*
   D. Protozoan:
      1. Toxoplasmosis
   E. Viral*:
      1. Cat-scratch disease
      2. Herpes simplex
      3. Infectious mononucleosis
      4. Lymphogranuloma venereum
      5. Ornithosis
      6. Psittacosis
III. Malignancy*:
   A. Hodgkin's disease
   B. Leukemia
   C. Postradiated pelvic cancer
IV. Miscellaneous:
   A. Behçet's disease

X-1 CONDITIONS ASSOCIATED WITH ERYTHEMA NODOSUM (CONTINUED)

    B. Inflammatory bowel disease:
        1. Ulcerative colitis.
        2. Crohn's disease*
    C. Pregnancy*
    D. Sarcoidosis

*Rare

Modified from: White JW Jr. Hurley H. In Moschella S, Hurley H, editors: *Dermatology*, ed 2. Philadelphia, 1985, W. B. Saunders, p. 465.

X-2 CAUSES OF ANHIDROSIS

   I. Neuropathic
    A. Hysteria
    B. Diseases or tumors of:
       1. Hypothalamus
       2. Pons
       3. Medulla
       4. Spinal cord
       5. Sympathetic nerves
  II. Sweat gland disturbances
    A. Congenital defects
       1. Generalized
       2. Localized
    B. Acquired defects
       1. Dermal diseases
       2. Drugs - anticholinergics
       3. Toxic chemicals
    C. Obstruction of sweat ducts
       1. Inflammatory or keratotic dermatoses
       2. Miliaria
 III. Idiopathic or indeterminate
    A. Newborn
    B. Local radiant heat or pressure
    C. Toxic
    D. Dehydration
    E. Systemic disease
    F. Franceschetti-Jadassohn syndrome
    G. Helweg-Larssen syndrome
    H. Fabry's disease

Modified from: Hurley H. In Moschella S, Hurley H, editors: *Dermatology*, ed 2. Philadelphia, 1985, W. B. Saunders, p. 1353.

X-3 SUSPECTED ETIOLOGIC FACTORS IN ERYTHEMA MULTIFORME

I. Infections:
   A. Herpes simplex
   B. Infectious mononucleosis
   C. Vaccinia
   D. Tuberculosis
   E. Tularemia
   F. Yersinia
   G. Histoplasmosis
II. Physical factors:
   A. X-ray therapy
III. Drugs:
   A. Anticonvulsants, especially hydantoins
   B. Barbiturates
   C. Sulfonamides, including hypoglycemics

*Modified from: Elias P, Fritsch P. In Fitzpatrick TB, Eisen AZ, Wolff K, Freedberg IM, Austen KF, editors: *Dermatology in general medicine*, ed 3. New York, 1987, McGraw-Hill, p. 556.

X-4 CLINICAL MANIFESTATIONS OF MASTOCYTOSIS

I. Cutaneous	Reddish-brown papules
	Flush
II. Cardiovascular	Tachycardia, hypotension, and syncope (rarely fatal)
III. Gastrointestinal	Nausea, vomiting, diarrhea (exacerbated by alcohol)
	Malabsorption (rare)
	Portal hypertension (rare)
IV. Bone	Pain
V. Neurologic	Neuropsychiatric symptoms (malaise, irritability)
VI. Respiratory	Rhinorrhea, wheezing (rare)
VII. Hematologic	Anemia, leukopenia, thrombo-cytopenia (rare)
	Eosinophilia
	Coagulopathies
	Leukemia (rare)

Source: Lewis R, Austen K. In Fitzpatrick TB, Eisen AZ, Wolff K, Freedberg IM, Austen KF, editors: *Dermatology in general medicine*, ed 3. New York, 1987, McGraw-Hill, p. 1900.

X-5 CLASSIFICATION OF CUTANEOUS SIGNS OF INTERNAL MALIGNANCY

I. Lesions secondary to the deposition of substances in the skin
   A. Icterus
   B. Melanosis
   C. Hemochromatosis
   D. Xanthomas
   E. Systemic amyloidosis

II. Vascular and blood abnormalities
   A. Flushing
   B. Palmar erythema
   C. Telangiectasia
   D. Purpura
   E. Vasculitis
   F. Cutaneous ischemia
   G. Thrombophlebitis

III. Bullous disorders
   A. Bullous pemphigoid
   B. Pemphigus vulgans
   C. Dermatitis herpetiformis
   D. Herpes gestationis
   E. Erythema multiforme
   F. Epidermolysis bullosa acquisita

IV. Infections and manifestations
   A. Herpes zoster
   B. Herpes simplex
   C. Bacterial infections
   D. Fungi and yeast infections
   E. Scabies

V. Disorders of keratinization
   *A. Acanthosis nigricans
   B. Acquired ichthyosis
   C. Palmar hyperkeratosis
   D. Erythroderma
   *E. Paraneoplastic acrokeratosis of Bazex

VI. Collagen-vascular disease
   A. Dermatomyositis
   B. Lupus erythematosus
   C. Progressive systemic sclerosis

VII. Skin tumors and internal malignant disease
   A. Muir-Torre syndrome
   B. Gardner's syndrome
   C. Cowden's disease
   D. Mucosal neuroma syndrome
   E. Neurofibromatosis

VIII. Hormone-related conditions

X-5 CLASSIFICATION OF CUTANEOUS SIGNS OF INTERNAL MALIGNANCY (CONTINUED)

IX. Disorders associated with primary skin cancer
    A. Nevoid basal cell carcinoma syndrome
    B. Arsenical manifestations

X. Various disorders associated with internal malignant disease
    A. Pruritus
   *B. Erythema gyratum repens
    C. Subcutaneous fat necrosis
   *D. Sweet's syndrome
   *E. Hypertrichosis lanuginosa acquisita
   *F. Necrolytic migratory erythema
    G. Clubbing
    H. Leukoderma
    I. Peutz-Jeghers syndrome
    J. Tuberous sclerosis
    K. Wiskott-Aldrich syndrome
    L. Multiple eruptive seborrheic keratoses
    M. Porphyria cutanea tarda
   *N. Paget's disease

XI. Direct tumor involvement in the skin

*definite associations

Modified from: Mclean D, Haynes H. In Fitzpatrick TB, Eisen AZ, Wolff K, Freedberg IM, Austen KF, editors: *Dermatology in general medicine*, ed 3. New York, 1987, McGraw-Hill, p. 1918.

X-6 DRUGS THAT CAUSE PRURITUS

I. Opiates and derivatives:
   A. Cocaine
   B. Morphine
   C. Butorphanol
II. Drug-induced pruritus via cholestasis:
   A. Phenothiazines
   B. Tolbutamide
   C. Erythromycin estolate
   D. Anabolic hormones
   E. Estrogens
   F. Progestins
   G. Testosterone
III. Aspirin
IV. Quinidine
V. Vitamin B complex
VI. Psoralen + UVA radiation (PUVA)
VII. Subclinical sensitivity to any drug

Modified from: Bernard J. In Fitzpatrick TB, Eisen AZ, Wolff K, Freedberg IM, Austen KF, editors: *Dermatology in general medicine,* ed 3. New York, 1987, McGraw-Hill, p. 81.

CHAPTER XI
ACQUIRED
IMMUNODEFICIENCY
SYNDROME (AIDS)

XI-1 DIAGNOSTIC CRITERIA FOR ACQUIRED IMMUNODEFICIENCY SYNDROME (AIDS)

I. Laboratory evidence for HIV infection
   A. Serum ELISA reactive for HIV antibody with subsequent HIV-antibody tests (Western blot) positive (for patients > 15 months old)
   B. Positive test for HIV serum antigen
   C. Positive HIV culture
   D. Positive result on any other highly specific test for HIV (DNA probe)

II. Indicator diseases diagnosed definitively without supporting laboratory evidence of HIV infection (cannot have other recognized causes of immunodeficiency)
   A. Candidiasis of esophagus, trachea, bronchi, or lungs
   B. Extrapulmonary cryptococcus
   C. Cryptosporidiosis with diarrhea > 1 month
   D. Cytomegalovirus disease of an organ other than liver, spleen, or lymph nodes (Patient > 1 month old)
   E. Herpes simplex virus causing mucocutaneous ulcer persisting longer than one month/ or bronchitis, pneumonitis, or esophagitis (any duration in patient older than one month.)
   F. Kaposi's sarcoma (patient < 60 years old)
   G. Primary lymphoma of brain (patient < 60 years old)
   H. Lymphoid interstitial pneumonia and/or pulmonary lymphoid hyperplasia (LIP/PLH complex) affecting child < 13 years old
   I. *Mycobacterium avium* complex or *M. kansasii* disease, disseminated
   J. *Pneumocystis carinii* pneumonia
   K. Progressive multifocal leukoencephalopathy
   L. Toxoplasmosis of the brain (patient > 1 month of age)

III. Indicator disease diagnosed definitively with laboratory evidence for HIV infection
   A. Bacterial infections, multiple or recurrent (any combination of at least two within a 2 year period):
      septicemia, pneumonia, meningitis, bone or joint, abscess of internal organ (excluding otitis media or superficial skin/mucosal abscess). (In a child < 13 years old)
   B. Disseminated coccidiomycosis
   C. HIV encephalopathy
   D. Disseminated histoplasmosis
   E. Isosporiasis with diarrhea > 1 month
   F. Kaposi's sarcoma
   G. Primary lymphoma of brain
   H. Non-Hodgkin's lymphoma of B-cell or unknown

XI-1 DIAGNOSTIC CRITERIA FOR ACQUIRED IMMUNODEFICIENCY SYNDROME (AIDS) (CONTINUED)

   immunologic phenotype (usually high grade)
   I. Disseminated mycobacterial disease
   J. Recurrent Salmonella sepsis
   K. HIV wasting syndrome
IV. Indicator diseases - diagnosed presumptively with laboratory evidence of HIV disease
   A. Esophageal Candidiasis
   B. Cytomegalovirus retinitis with loss of vision
   C. Kaposi's sarcoma
   D. Lymphoid interstitial pneumonia and/or pulmonary lymphoid hyperplasia affecting a child < 13 years of age
   E. Disseminated mycobacterial disease
   F. Pneumocystis pneumonia
   G. Toxoplasmosis of the brain (patient > 1 month old)
V. Other
   Any of the above diseases diagnosed definitively; with negative:
   A. Laboratory evidence of HIV infection *and* CD_4 lymphocyte count < 400 mm³
   B. CD_4 count < 200 mm³ and laboratory evidence of HIV infection (proposed)

Adapted from: *MMWR* 36 (15):1S-15S, 1987.

XI-2 RELATION OF CLINICAL MANIFESTATIONS TO CD4 COUNT IN HIV-INFECTED PATIENTS

Circulating CD4 Count at Time of Initial Susceptibility

	> 500	500-200	< 200	< 50
Asymptomatic / Kaposi Sarcoma	• •			
Fever, Sweats, Weight Loss / Hairy Leukoplakia / Oral, Esophageal Candida / Tuberculosis		• • • •		
Pneumocystosis / Cryptococcosis / Dementia			• • •	
Toxoplasmosis / Mycobacterium A/I / CMV / Death				• • • •

From: Shelhamer JH, et al. *Ann Intern Med* 117(5):419, 1992.

XI-3 RENAL SYNDROMES IN PATIENTS WITH HIV INFECTION

I. Coincidental renal syndromes and HIV
  A. Acute renal failure (ARF)
    1. Acute tubular necrosis from hypovolemic, anoxic and toxic injuries
    2. Allergic interstitial nephritis from drugs
    3. Azotemia from nonsteroidal antiinflammatory drugs
    4. Renal failure from massive proteinuria and severe hypoalbuminemia (intrarenal edema)
    5. Postinfectious immune complex glomerulonephritis
    6. Sulfadiazine and acyclovir crystal induced renal failure
    7. Plasmacytic interstitial nephritis
    8. Hemolytic uremic syndrome
  B. Acid-base and fluid-electrolyte derangements
    1. Hypo- and hypernatremia
    2. Inappropriate secretion of antidiuretic hormone (ADH)
    3. Hypo- and hyperkalemia
    4. Type IV renal tubular acidosis (hyporeninemic hypoaldosteronism)
    5. Metabolic alkalosis
    6. Hypomagnesemia
    7. Hypouricemia
  C. Infections in the kidney
    1. Microabscesses from bacterial infections (*Staphylococcus aureus*)
    2. Tuberculosis of the kidney (both typical and atypical mycobacterium)
    3. Cytomegalovirus infection
    4. Candida, cryptococcal, aspergillus and other fungal infections
  D. Infiltrations in the kidney
    1. Lymphoma of the kidney
    2. Kaposi's sarcoma
    3. Amyloidosis of the kidney
    4. Calcifications of the kidney
II. Specific (?) renal disorder; HIV-associated nephropathy
  A. Focal and segmental glomerulosclerosis
  B. Other forms of glomerulonephritis
III. Renal disease occurring in HIV seropositive patients
  A. Heroin-associated nephropathy
  B. Diabetic glomerulosclerosis, polycystic kidney disease, etc.
  C. Obstructive uropathy
IV. Superimposed HIV infection in those with renal replacement therapy

XI-3 RENAL SYNDROMES IN PATIENTS WITH HIV INFECTION (CONTINUED)

A. Maintenance dialysis patients acquiring HIV from blood transfusions, intravenous drug abuse, and sexual contacts

B. Renal transplant recipients developing HIV infection through renal allograft, blood transfusions, intravenous drug abuse, and sexual contacts

Modified from: Rao TK. Human immunodeficiency virus associated nephropathy. *Ann Rev Med* 1991. 42:391-401.

XI-4 MAJOR ENDOCRINE COMPLICATIONS IN ACQUIRED IMMUNODEFICIENCY SYNDROMES

Gland	Complication	Most Likely Causes
Adrenal	Cortisol and aldosterone deficiency	Opportunistic infection or ketoconazole
Pituitary	Syndrome of inappropriate anti-diuretic hormone (SIADH)	Pulmonary or central nervous system infection or drugs
Thyroid	Euthyroid sick	Systemic illness
Pancreatic islets	Hypoglycemia	Pentamidine, inanition, or sepsis
Testis	Hypogonadism	Hypothalamic deficiency secondary to systemic illness or ketoconazole
	Gynecomastia	Ketoconazole
Parathyroid	Hypocalcemia	Systemic illness or hypomagnesemia

Aron DC. Endocrine complications of the Acquired Immunodeficiency Syndrome. *Arch Intern Med* 149:330, 1989.

XI-5 GASTROINTESTINAL MANIFESTATIONS OF AIDS*

I. Mouth
   A. Candidiasis
   B. Aphthous ulcers
   C. Hairy leukoplakia
II. Esophagus
   A. Candidiasis
   B. CMV infection
   C. Herpes simplex
III. Liver and Biliary Tract
   A. Viral hepatitis *(types A, B, and C)
   B. Chronic active hepatitis
   C. CMV hepatitis
   D. Hepatic granulomas (e.g., fungal, drug-induced)
   E. Alcoholic hepatitis
   F. Steatosis
   G. Neoplasia (lymphoma)
   H. Sclerosing cholangitis (CMV, cryptosporidiosis)
   I. Ampullary stenosis
IV. Small Bowel
   A. CMV infection
   B. Cryptosporidiosis
   C. Giardiasis
   D. *Isopora belli* infection
   E. Microsporidiosis
   F. MAI infection
   G. "AIDS enteropathy"

XI-6 GASTROINTESTINAL PATHOGENS IN HIV-INFECTED PATIENTS*

Organ	Pathogens
Esophagus	*Candida albicans;* herpes simplex virus; cytomegalovirus
Stomach	Cytomegalovirus; *Mycobacterium avium-intracellulare*
Small intestine	*Cryptosporidium; Microsporidium; Isospora belli; Mycobacterium avium-intracellulare; Salmonella* species; *Campylobacter jejuni*
Colon	Cytomegalovirus; *Chlamydia trachomatis; Cryptosporidium; Mycobacterium avium-intracellulare;* amebiasis; candidiasis; *Shigella flexneri; Clostridium difficile; Campylobacter jejuni; Histoplasma capsulatum;* adenovirus; herpes simplex virus (rectum); gonorrhea (proctitis); syphilis (proctitis)

*HIV = human immunodeficiency virus.

Modified from: Smith PD, et al. *Ann Intern Med* 116(1):64, 1992.

XI-7 RHEUMATOLOGIC MANIFESTATIONS OF INFECTION WITH HUMAN IMMUNODEFICIENCY VIRUS (HIV)

I. Arthritis
   A. The Reiter syndrome and other reactive arthritides
   B. Psoriatic arthritis
   C. Septic arthritis caused by opportunistic organisms
   D. HIV-associated arthritis
II. Arthralgia
III. Myopathies
   A. Polymyositis
   B. Zidovudine-induced myositis
   C. Necrotizing, noninflammatory myopathy
   D. Pyomyositis
   E. Infectious myositis with opportunistic organisms
   F. Nemaline (rod) myopathy
   G. Myositis ossificans
   H. Subclinical myopathy
IV. Vasculitis
   A. Necrotizing vasculitis
   B. Eosinophilic vasculitis
   C. Isolated granulomatous angiitis of the central nervous system
   D. Leukocytoclastic vasculitis
   E. Lymphomatoid granulomatosis
   F. The sicca syndrome

From: Kaye BR. *Ann Intern Med* 111(2):159, 1989.

XI-8 AIDS ASSOCIATED HEMATOLOGIC DISORDERS

I. Anemia (70%)
  A. Marrow infiltration
    1. Infection: MAI, CMV, Cryptococcus, Histoplasmosis
    2. Lymphoma
  B. GI blood loss (Kaposi's sarcoma)
  C. Antierythrocyte antibodies (espescially anti-I)
  D. Myelosuppression due to drugs: AZT, gancyclovir, pentamidine, trimethoprim-sulfamethoxazole, acyclovir

II. Thrombocytopenia (40%)
  A. Immune-mediated destruction (ITP)
  B. Impaired synthesis — marrow infiltration
  C. HUS/TTP-like syndromes
  D. Drugs: e.g., AZT

III. Granulocytopenia (50%)

IV. Lymphopenic (70%)

V. Coagulation abnormalities
  A. Antiphospholipid antibody with elevated PTT

Adapted from: Scadden D, Zon L, Groopman J. Pathophysiology: management of HIV-associated hematologic disorders. *Blood*, 74(5):1455-1461, October, 1989.

XI-9 MUCOCUTANEOUS MANIFESTATIONS IN AIDS

I. Skin
   A. Infections
      1. Exaggerated scabies
      2. Herpes zoster (dermatomal or disseminated)
      3. Molluscum contagiosum
      4. Herpes simplex
      5. Dermatophytosis
      6. Cat-scratch disease
      7. Cutaneous cryptococcosis
   B. Granuloma annulare
   C. Kaposi's sarcoma
   D. Psoriatic exacerbation
   E. Inflammatory seborrheic dermatitis
   F. Ichthyosis
   G. Xerosis
   H. Papulonodular demodicidosis
   I. Bacillary epithelial angiomatosis
II. Hair
   A. Alopecia areata
   B. AIDS trichopathy
III. Nails
   A. Yellow nail syndrome
   B. Purple nail bands due to AZT
IV. Mouth
   A. Thrush
   B. Kaposi's sarcoma
   C. Hairy leukoplakia

Modified from: Orkin M, Maibach HE, Dahl MV. *Dermatology*, Norwalk, Conn., 1991, Appleton & Lange, p.145.

XI-10 PULMONARY COMPLICATIONS OF HIV INFECTION

I. Infections
- A. Viruses
    1. Cytomegalovirus
    2. Herpes simplex virus
    3. Varicella-zoster virus
    4. Epstein-Barr virus?
    5. Human immunodeficiency virus?
- B. Bacteria
    1. Pyogenic organisms (especially *Streptococcus pneumoniae, Hemophilus influenzae*)
    2. *Mycobacterium tuberculosis*
    3. *Mycobacterium avium* complex
    4. Other nontuberculous mycobacteria
    5. *Rhodococcus equi*
- C. Fungi
    1. *Histoplasma capsulatum*
    2. *Coccidioides immitis*
    3. *Cryptococcus neoformans*
    4. *Candida* species
    5. *Aspergillus* species
- D. Parasites
    1. *Pneumocystis carinii*
    2. *Toxoplasma gondii*
    3. Cryptosporidia
    4. *Strongyloides stercoralis*

V. Malignancies
- A. Kaposi's sarcoma
- B. Non-Hodgkin's lymphoma

VI. Interstitial pneumonias
- A. Lymphocytic interstitial pneumonitis
- B. Nonspecific interstitial pneumonitis
- C. Drug-induced reactions

VII. Other
- A. Adult respiratory distress syndrome
- B. Secondary alveolar proteinosis

Murray J, Mills J. Pulmonary infectious complication of human immunodeficiency virus infection. *Am Rev Respir Dis* 141:1357, 1990.

XI-11 NEUROLOGIC PROBLEMS IN AIDS PATIENTS

I. Infections
   A. Central nervous system
      1. Toxoplasmosis
      2. Cryptococcosis
      3. Herpes simplex
      4. Cytomegalovirus (encephalitis, retinitis)
      5. Neurosyphilis
      6. Progressive multifocal leukoencephalopathy
      7. Candidiasis
      8. Nocardiosis
      9. Coccidiosis
      10. Tuberculosis
      11. Mycobacterium avium-intracellulare
      12. Varicella-zoster encephalitis
   B. Peripheral nervous system
      1. Herpes zoster
      2. Cytomegalovirus polyradiculopathy
      3. HIV polyneuritis
II. Noninfectious
   A. Central nervous system
      1. HIV dementia
      2. Vacuolar myelopathy
      3. Lymphoma
      4. Kaposi's sarcoma
   B. Peripheral nervous system
      1. Sensory neuropathy
      2. Inflammatory demyelinating neuropathy
      3. Mononeuritis multiplex
      4. Polymyositis and other myopathies

XI-12 CANCERS IN THE HIV EPIDEMIC

I. Incidence increased:
   A. Kaposi's sarcoma
   B. CNS non-Hodgkin's lymphoma
   C. Peripheral non-Hodgkin's lymphoma
   D. Cervical carcinoma

II. Cases reported:
   A. Hodgkin's lymphoma
   B. Squamous carcinoma
   C. Small cell carcinoma
   D. Testicular cancer
   E. Basal cell cancer
   F. Melanoma

III. Anticipated relationship:
   A. Hepatocellular carcinoma

Reference: Chaisson R Volberding P. Clinical manifestations of HIV infection. In: Mandell GL, Douglas G Jr, Bennett JE, editors: *Principles and practice of infectious diseases*, 3rd Edition, 1985, Churchill Livingstone, New York, p. 1085.

INDEX

A

Abcess
  of brain, mortality in 177
  lung, etiologic classification,
    235
Acanthocytes 139
  Achalasia, 79 (See also
    Esophagus)
Achalasia 83
Acidosis
  metabolic, differential
    diagnosis 200
      with increased anion gap
        199
      with low anion gap 200
      with normal anion gap
        (hyperchloremic) 200
  renal tubular acidosis (RTA),
    differential diagnosis
      type I 204
      type II 206
      type IV 207
  respiratory
    differential diagnosis 226
  rules of thumb for bedside
    interpretation 228
Acquired immunodeficiency
  syndrome (AIDS)

    associated hematologic
      disorders 309
  cancers in the HIV
    epidemic 313
  diagnostic criteria 300
  endocrine complications 305
  gastrointestinal
    manifestations 306
  gastrointestinal
    pathogens 307
  mucocutaneous
    manifestations 310
  neurologic problems 312
  pulmonary complications 311
  relation of clinical
    manifestations to CD4
      count 302
  renal syndromes 303
  rheumatologic
    manifestations 308
Acromegaly (See Pituitary:
  Growth hormone)
Acute confusional states:
  classification 287
Addison's disease:
  clinical features 55
Adrenal gland
  adrenal cortical
    insufficiency 54

Addison's disease 55
  corticosteroid therapy 77
  Cushing's syndrome 55
    clinical features 56
  primary aldosteronism 57
  secondary hyperaldosteronism:
    classification 58
Alcoholism
  alcoholic hepatitis
    clinical and histological
      features 100
  alcoholic liver disease
    spectrum 100
  chronic, diagnosis 99
Aldosterone
  primary aldosteronism 67
  secondary hyperaldosteronism
    classification 58
Alkalosis
  bedside interpretation 228
  differential diagnosis
    metabolic 198
    respiratory 227
Allergic bronchopolmonary
  aspergillosis:
    diagnostic criteria 253
Alveolor
  hyperventilation, differential
    diagnosis 230
  hyperventilation, chronic,
    differential diagnosis 248
Amenorrhea: causes 72
Anaerobic infections 188
Anemia
  aplastic
    differential diagnosis 138
  hemolytic 135
  macrocytic 133
  microcytic-hypochromic 133
  normochromic-
    normocytic 132
  pancytopenia 137
Anesthetics: in hepatic
  encephalopathy 108-109
Angiitis: in eosinophilic lung
  disease 243

Angiography
  in liver hyperplasia and
    adenoma 114-115
Anhidrosis: causes 293
Anion gap (See Acidosis,
  metabolic)
Ankylosing spondylitis
  diagnostic criteria 271
Anorexia nervosa 87
Antiarrhythmic drugs:
  classification by action
    mechanism 32
Antibiotic associated
  pseudomembranous colitis
    186
Antibody
  autoantibodies in SLE 264
  in acquired immunodeficiency
    syndrome 300-301
Anticoagulation: risk factors 15
Antidiuresis: inappropriate
  syndrome 47-48
Antigens: and autoantibodies
  in SLE 264
Antineoplastic chemotherapy:
  responses to 160-161
Aortic regurgitation: causes 6
Arrhythmias. See Heart:
  Arrhythmias
Arteritis: giant-cell 277
Arthritis
  autoantibodies in rheumatic
    diseases
      disease associations
        and molecular
        identification 278
  gouty arthritis
    diagnostic criteria 272
  inflammatory monoarthritis
    differential diagnosis 273
  monoarthritis, inflammatory,
    differential diagnosis 273
  psoriatic arthritis
    provisional diagnostic
      criteria 272

rheumatoid factor
  differential diagnosis of
    positive blood test 275
Arthropathy: sarcoid 274
Ascites
  differential diagnosis 109-110
  pancreatic 122
Aseptic meningitis 285
Aspergillosis: allergic
  bronchopulmonary, diagnostic
    criteria 253
Atherogenicity: of lipoprotein
  particles 74
Atherosclerotic heart disease
  (AHD): risk factors 8
Atrial
  fibrillation, causes 7
  flutter, causes 7
  septal defect, classification 7
Autoantibodies: in SLE 264
Autoimmunity: hypersensitivity of,
  and pericarditis 24
Azotemia 108

B

Bacteremia: gram-negative rod,
  outcome 181
Bacteria
  meningitis due to 285
  overgrowth syndromes 90
Basophilia: differential diagnosis
  142
Basophilic stippling 143
B-cell deficiency syndrome 242
Behçet's syndrome
  diagnosis 267
Bile salt: in malabsorption
  syndrome 88
Biliary cirrhosis: primary 107
Binet classification: of lymphocytic
  leukemia 148
Bleeding (See Gastrointestinal
  hemorrhage)
Blood
  abnormalities in internal
    cancer 295-196

multiple myeloma
  diagnostic criteria 148
  renal and electrolyte
    disorders in 150
  staging 149
myelodysplastic
  syndromes 147
myeloproliferative
  syndromes 147
peripheral smear -
  abnormalities
    differential diagnosis 143
  to brain, altered state 21-22
  test, positive, for rheumatoid
    factor 275
  thrombosis
    predisposing risk
      factors 169
Bone
  cancers metastatic to 159
  marrow (See Marrow)
  in mastocytosis 294
Botulism: food poisoning
  secondary to 185
Bowel
  bacterial proliferation in, in
    malabsorption syndrome
    88-89
  irritable bowel syndrome,
    diagnosis 94
Bradyarrhythmia 21
Brain
  abscess, mortality in 180
  blood to, altered state 21
Breast cancer, survival in 156
Bronchi: metastases to 240
Bronchiectasis: differential
  diagnosis 255
Bronchogenic carcinoma:
  paraneoplastic syndromes in
    256-257
Bronchopulmonary
  aspergillosis: allergic,
    diagnostic criteria 253
Bullous disorders: in internal
  cancer 295-296

C

Calcium stones
    risk factors 71
Cancer
    antineoplastic chemotherapy,
        responses to 160-61
    breast, survival in 156
    colon, risk factors for
        developing 98
    in erythema nodosum 293
    hypercalcemia in, hormonal
        basis of 159
    hyponatremia in, causes 156
    internal, cutaneous signs of,
        classification 295-196
    kidney in, complications 222
    lung, TNM nomenclature
        in 157
    metastatic
        to bone 159
        to lung, differential
            diagnosis 255
    myelotoxicity of therapy
        160-161
    in pericardial effusions 158
    in peritoneal effusions 158
    in pleural effusion,
        malignant 158
    skin 296
Cardiac (See Heart)
Cardiogenic shock 10
Cardiomyopathy congestive 13
    etiologic classification 16-17
Cardiovascular
    disorders
        in hemoptysis 235
        in malabsorption
            syndrome 88-89
        in mastocytosis 295-296
        in uremia 224-225
        risk in patients considered
            for surgery 31
Cauda equina syndrome 163
Celiac sprue
    diagnosis 90

Cell(s)
    B-cell deficiency syndrome 242
    germ cell tumors 256-257
    giant-cell arteritis 277
    target 143
    T-cell deficiency syndrome 242
    Central nervous system
        in AIDS 312
    in hyperprolactinemia 45
    in hypoventilation, chronic
        alveolar 248
    in pancreatitis, acute 122
    in SIADH 47
Cerebrospinal fluid: glucose
    decrease 312
Chemicals: liver morphology due
    to 118
Chemotherapy
    antineoplastic, responses to
        160-161
DNA metabolism interfered with
    in 133
Chest
    pain in pulmonary embolism
        249
    radiography (See Radiography,
        chest)
    wall disease in respiratory
        failure 245
Cholangitis: sclerosing,
    primary 128
Cholecystectomy: post
    cholecystectomy syndrome
    124
Cholesterol gallstone:
    predisposing factors 129
Chronic fatigue syndrome
    diagnostic criteria 194
Circulatory deficiency 21-22
Cirrhosis: biliary, primary 107
Clubbing of digits, differential
    diagnosis 234
Colitis
    antibiotic associated
        pseudomembranous 186
    ulcerative idiopathic 92

systemic manifestations 93
vs. granulomatous colitis 92
Collagen-vascular disease: in
internal cancer 295-296
Colon cancer: risk factors for
developing 98
Coma
classification 284
differential diagnosis 284
Completement deficiency
syndrome 242
Confusional states: classification
287-288
Conjunctivitis: in Reiter's
syndrome 271
Conn's Syndrome. See Adrenal
gland: Primary aldosteronism
Connective tissue disorders
in FUO 172-173
in Raynaud's phenomenon 265
Consciousness: episodic
disturbances 21-22
Constipation: in hepatic
encephalopathy 108
Cor pulmonale: chronic,
respiratory disorders
predisposing to 28
Corticosteroids: complications
of 77-78
Cough: with negative chest
radiography, differential
diagnosis 239
CPPD crystal deposition
putative associations 279
Cryoglobulinemia 276
Crystal
deposition, CPPD, putative
associations 279
induced inflammatory
monoarthritis 273
Cushing's syndrome 55
clinical features 56
Cutaneous (See Skin)
Cyanosis: causes 154
Cytomegalovirus
mononucleosis: features 179

D

Death
in brain abscess 180
sudden, nontraumatic,
causes 14
Dehydration: in oliguria 213
Delirium: classification 287-288
Delta agent. 127
Dementia: classification 287
Depression: secondary
causes 289
Diabetes insipidus
central, differential diagnosis
218-219
nephrogenic, differential
diagnosis 217-218
Diabetes mellitus.
classification 61
ketoacidosis of, precipitating
factors 62
Dialysis: renal, lung
complications 229
Diarrhea
classification 95-97
diagnosis 95-97
management 95-97
Digestion: in malabsorption
syndrome 88-89
Digitalis
intoxication 30
toxic dose
risk factors 30
diagnosis 30
Digits: clubbing of, differential
diagnosis 284
Diuretics: in hepatic
encephalopathy 108
DNA metabolism: interfered with
by chemotheraphy 133
Drug(s)
antiarrhythmic, classification
by action mechanism 32
in ARDS 251
in depression 289
in erythema
multiforme 294

nodosum 292-294
  liver morphology due to 118
  neutropenia 139
  pruritus due to 297
  in Raynaud's phenomenon 265
  in tuberculosis 190-191
Duodenal ulcer: refractory,
  differential diagnosis 85

E

ECG exercise tests
  purpose 9
Edema: generalized, conditions
  leading to 223
Electrical stimulation:
  endocardial 34-35
Electrocardiography continuous,
  long-term indications 33
  exercise tests, purposes of 9
  pseudoinfarction, patterns 13
  in pulmonary embolism 250
Electrolyte disturbances
  differential diagnosis
    hyperkalemia 202
    hypernatremia 203
    hypokalemia 201
    hyponatremia 204
  in diabetes insipidus
    nephrogenic 217-218
  in gastric emptying,
    delayed 86-87
  in myeloma, multiple 150
  in uremia 224-225
Electrophysiological studies:
  indications 34-35
Embolism, pulmonary
angiographically documented,
  symptoms and signs 249
ECG changes in 250
Empty sella syndrome: features
  associated with 46
Encephalitis-aseptic
  meningitis 285
Encephalopathy: hepatic,
  precipitating causes 108-109
Endobronchial metastases 255

Endocardial electrical stimulation
  34-35
Encodrine
  disorders
    in depression 289
    in malabsorption
      syndrome 88-89
    in uremia 224-225
  hypertension 19-20
  multiple endocrine neoplasia
    syndrome 168
Encocrinopathy
  in anemia 132
  in hypercalcemia 66
Enteritis, regional
  differential diagnosis 91
  systemic manifestations 93
Environmental exposure: in
  Raynaud's phenomenon 265
Eosinophilia:
  differential diagnosis 141
Eosinophilic lung disease:
  differential diagnosis 243
Eosinophilia: differential
  diagnosis 141
Eosinophilic lung disease:
  differential diagnosis 243
Erectile impotence:
  organic causes 75
Erythema
  multiform, suspected etiologic
    factors 294
  nodosum, conditions
    associated with 292-93
Erythrocytes
  erythrocytosis
    differential diagnosis 145
  glycolytic enzyme
    deficiency 135
  membrane defects 135
  nucleotide metabolism
    abnormalities 135
  polycythemia vera
    diagnostic criteria 146
Erythrocytosis: differential
  diagnosis 145

Esophagus
   achalasia 83
   esophageal motility disorders
      classification 82
   lesions, primary 256
   motility disorders,
      classification 82
Ethambutol: in tuberculosis,
   dosages 190-191
Exercise tests: ECG,
   purposes of 9
Extracellular fluid: in
   hyponatremia 204

F

Faintness: causes 21
Fanconi's syndrome 220-221
Fat necrosis: in acute
   pancreatitis 122-123
Fever
   Q, extrapulmonary
      manifestations 177
   after renal transplant 260
   rheumatic, Jones criteria 5
   of unknown origin, etiology,
      172-173
Fibrillation: atrial, causes 7
Fibromyalgia
   American College of
      Rheumatology 1990
      criteria 284
Fluid disturbances: in uremia
   224-225
Folate deficiency 133-135
Food poisoning: secondary to
   botulism 185
FUO: etiology 172-173

G

Galactorrhea: physiological
   classification 47
Gallstone
   cholesterol, predisposing
      factors 129

   pigment, predisposing
      factors 129
Gastric emptying: delayed 86-87
Gastrointestinal disease
   bacterial overgrowth
      syndrome 90
   chronic diarrheal disorders
      classification, diagnosis and
         management 95
   colon cancer: risk factors 98
   digital clubbing in 234
   exocrine pancreatic
      insufficiency (EPI):
         diagnosis 124
   granulomatous colitis
      differential diagnosis 92
   irritable bowel syndrome
      diagnosis 94
   malabsorption syndrome
      classification 88
   malnutrition
      criteria for assessing
         severity 125
   mastocytosis 295-296
   pancreatic exocrine
      insufficiency
         causes 119
   regional enteritis
      systemic manifestations 93
   ulcerative colitis (UC)
      systemic manifestations 93
   ulcerative colitis - idiopathic
      differential diagnosis 92
Genetic abnormalities: in
   malabsorption syndrome
   88-89
Genetics
   in hemolytic anemia 135
   in nephrotic syndrome
   214-216
Genitourinary tuberculosis:
   clinical features 173
Germ cell tumors 256
Giant-cell arteritis 277
Globin structural defects 135
Glomerular disease 136
Glomerulonephritis 208

acute, differential diagnosis 214

Glucose
cerebrospinal fluid, decrease in 290
in synovial fluid 280-281

Glutathione metabolism 135-136

Goiter 49

Gonococcal infection: spectrum of 184

Gout
hyperuricemia differential diagnosis 220

Gouty arthritis:
diagnostic criteria 272

Graft-vs.-host disease: clinical features 162

Granulomatosis: in eosinophilic lung disease 243

Granulomatous colitis 92
liver disease 126

Gynecomastia
differential diagnosis 73

H

Heart
antiarrhythmic drugs
mechanism of action 32
arrhythmias
atrial fibrillation 7
atrial flutter 7
atherosclerotic,
risk factors for 8
cardiac tamponade
causes 27
cardiomyopathies
etiologic classification 16
congenital defects
atrial septal defects 7
congestive heart failure
reversible causes 18
congestive heart failure (CHF)
causes 17
cor pulmonale
risk factors 28
digital clubbing in 234

endocardial electrical stimulation 34
endocarditis - bacterial prophylaxis 40
ischemic, prognostic determinants 12
murmurs
classification of continuous 4
innocent murmurs 2
mechanisms of continuous 4
myocardial infarction - acute complications 18
mycoplasma pneumoniae infection 176
output reduction 21
pacemaker
NBG code 36
pericarditis
causes of chronic constrictive 24
classification 23
clinical features of constrictive 25
psittacosis 177
risk in patients considered for surgery 31
sounds - second heart sound
causes of splitting 2
causes of single second heart sound 3
sudden death 14
tamponade, common etiologies 27
valves
aortic regurgitation 6
mitral regurgitation 5
mitral stenosis 8
pulmonary valve insufficiency 29
tricuspid regurgitation 7

Hematologic disorders
in ARDS 251
in basophilia 142
in mastocytosis 294

in neutropenia 139
in Raynaud's phenomenon 265
in SLE 264
in splenomegaly 151
in uremia 224-225
Hemochromatosis: idiopathic,
clinical features 113
Hemoglobin abnormalities:
in cyanosis 154
Hemolytic anemia:
differential diagnosis 135-136
Hemoptysis 235
Hemmorhage
(See Gastrointestinal
hemmorhage)
Hepatic (See Liver)
Hepatitis
A 101
alcoholic features 100-101
B 103-105
diagnosis 104
epidemiology 103
immunology of 103
infection, spectrum of
responses in 104
serologic abnormalities in,
interpretation of 105
C 102
non-A, non-B 102
Hepatoma: clinical features 116
Hilar enlargement
bilateral, differential
diagnosis 240
unilateral, differential
diagnosis 240
Hirsutism: causes in females 71
Histoplasmosis: clinical
phulmonary syndromes of 175
HIV infection 300-313
Hodgkin's disease:
histopathologic classification
164
"Honeycomb" lung 241
Hormone(s)
antidiuretic, inappropriate,
syndrome 47-48

in hypercalcemia of cancer 159
TSH 49
Howell-Jolly bodies 143-144
Hypercalcemia: conditions 66
Hyperchloremic acidosis
(See Acid-base disturbances:
Metabolic acidosis with normal
anion gap)
Hyperlactemia. See Lactic acid
Hyperlipidemia
atherogenicity of individual
lipoproteins 74
classification based on
lipoprotein
concentrations 74
primary vs secondary 75
Hypertension
prognosis 20
pulmonary
risk factors 28
types 19
Hyperuricemia. See Gout:
Hyperuricemia
Hypoalbuminemia
differential diagnosis 125
Hypocalcemia
nonparathyroid hypocalcemia
conditions 67
osteomalacia
classification 68
osteoporosis
classification 70
rickets
classification 68
Hypoglycemia: fasting, major
causes 63
Hypoglycorrhachia
causes 290
Hyponatremia
in cancer, causes 156
differential diagnosis 204
Hypoparathyroidism 67
Hypophosphatemia
causes 77
Hypopopituitarism: disorders
associated with 44-45

Hypothyroidism
    causes 50
    clinical features 50
Hypouricemia
    differential diagnosis 220
Hypoventilation: alveolar, chronic,
    differential diagnosis 248
Hypovolemia 21

I

Immune
    deficiency syndrome (See
        acquired immunodeficiency
        syndrome (AIDS)
Immune system
    graft-versus-host disease
        clinical features 162
Immunocompromised hoses 174
    lung infections in 175
Immunohemolytic anemia
    135-136
Immunologic
    disorder
        in SLE 264
        in uremia 224
        factors in splenomegaly
        151
Immunology
    of hepatitis B 103
Impotence: erectile, organic
    causes 75-76
Infarction
    type in as is myocardial 151
    pseudoinfarction ECG
        patterns 13
Infectious diseases
    in AIDS 300-311
    anaerobic infections 188
    arthritis, due to 273
    bacteremia
        risk factors affecting
        outcome 181
    botulism
        clinical features 185
    brain abscess
        mortality factors 180

cancer, internal 295
cytomegalovirus
    mononucleosis:
    clinical and laboratory
        features 179
erythema
    multiforme 294
    nodosum 292
fever of unknown origin (FUO)
    disease states causing
    FUO 172
gonococcal infections
    spectrum of 184
histoplasmosis
    pulmonary syndromes 175
immunocompromised hosts
    classification 174
legionella
    features 178
listeria monocytogenes
    infections 189
lung (See Lung, infection)
Lyme disease
    manifestations 192
mycoplasma pneumoniae
    extrapulmonary
        manifestations 176
nontuberculosis mycobacterial
    disease
        diagnostic criteria in
        nonimmunocompromised
        hosts 174
osteomyelitis
    major types 182
pneumonococcal
    pneumonia. See Pulmonary
    diseases
psittacosis
    extrapulmonary
        manifestations 177
psuedomembranous colitis
    antibiotic-associated 186
pulmonary infections
    immunocompromised
        patients 175

Q fever
extrapulmonary
manifestations 177
toxic shock syndrome 187
tuberculosis
classification 173
effective drug
regimens 190
genitourinary - clinical
features 173
Infestations: in internal
cancer 295
Inflammatory monoarthritis:
differential diagnosis 273
Inflammatory myopathies
diagnostic criteria 268
Insulin resistant states 64
Interstitial (See Lung disease,
interstitial)
Intestine (See Gastrointestinal)
Intoxication: digitalis 30
Iron
deficiency anemia 133
storage disease, differential
diagnosis 113
Irritable bowel syndrome:
diagnosis 94
Ischemic heart disease
prognostic determinants 12
Isoniazid: in tuberculosis,
dosages 190

J

Jaundice: postoperative 111
Jones criteria:
in rheumatic fever 5

K

Karnofsky scale 167
Ketoacidosis: diabetic,
precipitating factors 62
Kidney
(See also Renal)
in cancer, complications 222
disease
in diabetes insipidus
217-218
edema due to,
generalized 223
in lupus erythematosis,
systemic 264
in myeloma, multiple 148
parenchymal, causing
kidney failure 208
tubulointerstitial 216
failure due to parenchymal
disease 208
function, acute deterioration,
differential diagnosis
208-209
in Mycoplasma pneumoniae
infection 176
necrosis 208-209
in psittacosis 177
tubular
acidosis (See Acidosis, renal
tubular)
disease 216
injury in oliguria 213
transport in hypouricemia
220-221

L

Lactic acid
hyperlactemia: causes 79
Legionella infection: features 178
Leukemia: chronic lymphocytic,
staging 148
Leukocytes
basophilia
differential diagnosis 142
chronic lymphocytic leukemia
staging 148
monocytosis
disorders associated
with 143
neutropenia
differential diagnosis 139
neutrophilia
differential diagnosis 140
in synovial fluid 280
polymorphonuclear 280

Lipoprotein
concentrations,
hyperlipidemia
classification based on 74
Listeria monocytogenes
infection 189
Liver
adenoma, characteristics of
114-115
alterations of hepatic
morphology: drug and
chemical induced 118
ascites
differential diagnosis 109
biliary disease
gallstone formation -
predisposing factors 129
postcholecystectomy
syndrome 124
primary sclerosis
cholangitis 128
chronic active liver disease
etiology and diagnosis 106
disease
alcoholic, spectrum of 100
chronic active, etiology and
diagnosis 106
granulomatous 126
in malabsorption
syndrome 88
encephalopathy, precipitating
causes 108-109
focal nodular hyperplasia
comparison of clinical,
radiologic, and
pathologic 114
fulminant hepatic failure
causes 130
granulomatous liver
disease 126
hepatic encephalopathy 108
common precipitating
causes 108
hepatitis B 103
delta agent 127
hepatitis C 102

hepatoma
clinical features 115
hyperplasia, focal nodular,
characteristics 114-115
idiopathic hemochromocytosis
clinical features 113
intrahepatic cholestasis
differential diagnosis 112
iron storage disease
differential diagnosis 113
liver cell adenoma
comparison of clinical,
radiologic, and
pathologic 114
morphology due to drugs and
chemicals 118
postoperative jaundice
causes and contributing
conditions 111
primary biliary cirrhosis 107
Wilson's disease
diagnosis 117
Lung
(See also Pulmonary)
abscess, etiologic
classification 252
cancer, TNM nomenclature
in 157
disease
digital clubbing in 234
eosinophilic, differential
diagnosis 243
interstitial, differential
diagnosis 244
interstitial, diffuse, drugs in
etiology of 261
in uremia 224
"honeycomb" 241
infection
in AIDS 311
in immunocompromised
hosts 175
infiltrates in renal
transplant 260
manifestations of rheumatoid
arthritis 258

metastases to, differential
diagnosis 256-257
microcysts 241
nodular, solitary
differential diagnosis 254
nonmalignant lesions
presenting as 254
in sudden death 14
syndromes of histoplasmosis,
clinical 175
tumors
digital clubbing in 234
hemoptysis in 235
Lupus erythematosus, systemic
autoantibodies in 278
diagnostic criteria 264
Lymph
node(s)
enlargement 256-257
status in breast cancer
survival 156
obstruction in
malabsorption syndrome
88
Lymphadenopathy: differential
diagnosis 152-153
Lymphangitic mestastses 255
Lymphatic system
lymphadenopathy
differential diagnosis 152
Lymphomas
Hodgkin's disease
Cotswold staging 164
nonhodgkin's lymphomas
working formulation 165

M

Macrocytic anemia: differential
diagnosis 133-135
Magnesium
hypomagnesemia
causes 60
magensium depletion
causes 60
Malabsorption syndromes:
classification 88-89

Malignancy (See Cancer)
Malnutrition
in neutropenia 139
severity, assessment
criteria 126
Marrow
failure in anemia 132
in pancytopenia 138
Mastocytosis
clinical manifestations 294
Mediastinal mass: differential
diagnosis 256-257
Medications (See Drugs)
Meningitis
differential diagnosis 285
Mesenchymal tumors 256-257
Metabolic
acidosis (See Acidosis,
metabolic)
alkalosis (See Alkalosis,
metabolic)
disorders
in depression 289
in malabsorption syndrome
88-89
in uremia 224-225
Metabolism
glutathione 135-136
Metastases
to bone, cancers causing 159
endobronchial 255
to lung, differential
diagnosis 255
lymphangitic 255
Microcysts: of lung 240
Mitral
regurgitation, causes 5-6
stenosis, complications 8
Monoarthritis: inflammatory,
differential diagnosis 273
Mononucleosis:
cytomegalovirus, features 179
Mortality
in brain abscess 180
sudden death, nontraumatic
causes 14

Mucosal lymphoma: in Kaposi's sarcoma 294

Multiple endocrine neoplasia syndrome 168

Multiple myeloma (See Blood)

Murmurs

    continuous

        mechanisms of 4

        thoracic, causes of 4

    innocent 2

        completely 2

        relatively 2

Muscle

    disturbances in uremia 224-225

    neuromuscular (See Neuromuscular)

Mycobacterial disease: nontuberculosis, diagnostic criteria 174

Mycoplasma pneumoniae: extrapulmonary manifestations 176

Myelodysplastic syndromes 147

Myeloma, multiple

    diagnostic criteria 148

    electrolyte disorders in 150

    renal disorders in 150

Myeloproliferative syndromes 147

Myelotoxicity: of cancer therapy 160-161

Myocardial infarction (MI)

    acute,

        potential life-threatening complications 18

    causes, nonatherosclerotic 11

    subsets, clinical and hemodynamic 10

    involvement in cardiomyopathy 167-17

    causes

        nonatherosclerotic 11

    clinical subsets 10

    hemodynamic subsets 10

    psuedoinfarction ECG patterns 13

N

Necrosis

    fat, in acute pancreatitis 119-120

    kidney 208-209

    in lung abscess 252

Neoplasia

    antineoplastic chemotherapy

        general response of various malignancies 160

    breast cancer

        survival factors 156

    cauda equina syndrome. See nervous system: Peripheral nerve disease

    hypercalcemia of malignancy

        etiologic factors 159

    hyponatremia in cancer patients

        causes 156

    internal malignancy

        classification of cutaneous signs 295

    lung cancer

        TMN nomenclature 157

    lymphomas. See Lymphomas

    malignant pericardial effusions

        most frequent neoplasms causing 158

    malignant pleural effusions

        Most frequent types 158

    metastases to bone

        cancers most likely 159

    metastatic epidural compression

        signs and symptoms 163

    multiple endocrine neoplasia syndrome 168

    paraneoplastic syndromes 155

    performance status of patient 167

    peritoneal effusions

        most frequent malignancies causing 158

radiation therapy
  long-term effects 161
tumors metastatic to the lungs
  differential diagnosis 255
Nephrogenic diabetes insipidus:
  differential diagnosis 217-218
Nephrolithiasis: differential
  diagnosis 220
Nephrology 198-231
Nephrotic syndrome: differential
  diagnosis 214-216
Nephrotoxins: major 212
Nervous system
  peripheral nerve disease
    cauda equina
      syndrome 163
Neurogenic disorders: in
  Raynaud's phenomenon 265
Neurologic disorders
  in AIDS 271
  in depression 289
  in hypertension 19-20
  in mastocytosis 294
  in SLE 264
Neurology 284-290
Neuromuscular disorders
  in bronchogenic carcinoma
    237
  in hypoventionation, chronic
    alveolar 248
  in uremia 224-225
Neuron:
  respiratory, depression 248
Neuropathy: peripheral,
  differential diagnosis 286
Neutropenia: differential
  diagnosis 139
Neutrophilia: differential
  diagnosis 140
Nitrofurantoin 243
Nutrition deficiency (See
  Malnutrition)

O

Obesity: classification 65
Occupational exposure: in
  Raynaud's phenomenon 265

Oliguria: dehydration vs. tubular
  injury in 213
Oncology 132-169
Opiates: causing pruritus 297
Organ system failure
  modified APACHE II
    criteria 262
Osteomalacia: classification 68-69
Osteomyelitis 182-183
Osteoporosis: classification 70

P

Pacemaker
  implanted, definite indications
    for 33
  modes, code for 36
Pain: chest, in pulmonary
  embolism 249
Pancreas
  acute pancreatitis
    causes 119
    complications 122
  ascites 119-120
  chronic pancreatitis
    complications 123
  diabetes mellitus
    classification 61
    insulin resistant states 64
    late complications 80
  diabetic ketoacidosis
    precipitating factors 62
  hypoglycemia
    causes of fasting
      hypoglycemia 63
  insufficiency, exocrine
    causes 119
    diagnosis 124
Pancreatic exocrine
  insufficiency (See
  Gastrointestinal)
Pancreatitis
  acute
    causes 119-121
    complications 122-123
    survival, factors adversely
      influencing 121
    chronic, complications 123

Pancytopenia: differential diagnosis 137
Paraneoplastic syndromes 155
Parasites: in eosinophilic lung disease 243
Parathyroid glands
hypoparathyroidism
causes 67
Pentose phosphate 135-136
Performance status: Karnofsky scale 167
Pericardial effusion etiology 26
malignant 158
Pericarditis
classification 23-24
constrictive
chronic, etiology 24
clinical features 24
Pericardium. See Heart
pericarcial effusion
causes 26
Peripheral neuropathies
differential diagnosis 286
Peripheral smear abnormalities: differential diagnosis 143-144
Peritoneal effusions
cancers in 158
Phagocyte deficiency syndrome 242
Phosphorus absorption: in hypophosphatemia 77
Pigment gallstone: predisposing factors 129
Pituitary
antiduiretic hormone
syndrome of inappropriate antidiuretic hormone (SIADH) 47
central diabetes insipidus
differential diagnosis 218
in galactorrhea 47
growth hormone
acromegaly 46
hyperprolactemia 45
neurogenic diabetes insipidus.

See Pituitary: Central diabetes insipidus
primary empty sella syndrome
clinical features 46
prolactin
galactorrhea 47
Pituitary gland
hypopituitarism
disorders associated with 44
Pleural disease
in respiratory failure 245
effusions
diagnosis, differential 237
exudative, criteria for 238
malignant 158
transudative,
criteria for 238
Pneumococcal pneumonia: prognostic indicators 252
Pneumoconiosis 240
Pneumonia: pneumococcal, prognostic indicators 252
Pneumothorax: differential diagnosis 241
Poisoning: food, secondary to botulism 185
Polyarteritis nodosa 277
Polycythemia 145
vera, diagnostic criteria 146
Polymorphonuclear leukocytes 280-281
Polymyalgia rheumatica 266
diagnostic criteria 266
differential diagnosis 266
Post cholecystectomy syndrome 124
Progressive systemic sclerosis. See Scleroderma
Prolactin 45
Pruritus: causative drugs 297
Pseudohyperkalemia 202
Pseudohypoaldosteronism 207
Psuedoinfarction: ECG patterns 13
Psittacosis: extrapulmonary manifestations 177

Psoriatic arthritis: provisional diagnostic criteria 272-273

Psychomotor underactivity: in confusional states 287-288

Pulmonary diseases
  differential diagnosis
    adult respiratory distress syndrome: clinical disorders associated with 251
    allergic bronchopulmonary aspergillosis: diagnostic criteria 253
    alveolar hyperventilation 247
    bronchiectasis 236
    chronic alveolar hypoventilation 248
    clubbing of the digits 234
    cough with negative chest x-ray 239
    eosiniphilic lung disease 243
    hemoptysis 235
    hilar enlargement 240
    mechanical ventilation guidelines for withdrawl 246
    pleural effusions 237
    evaluation 238
    pneumonococcal pneumonia prognostic indicators 252
    pneumothorax 241
    pulmonary emboli symptoms and signs 249
    pulmonary embolism ECG changes 250
    pulmonary interstitial disease 244
    pulmonary manifestations vascular collagen diseases 258
    pulmonary parenchymal injury: drugs implicated in the etiology 261
    pulmonary renal syndromes 259
    recurrent pulmonary infection associated with immunodeficiency syndromes other than HIV-related 242
    respiratory failure 245
    solitary pulmonary nodules 254

Pulmonary disorders
  mediastinal mass 256

Purpura: thrombotic thrombocytopenic, diagnostic criteria 150

Pyloric outlet obstruction: causing delayed gastric emptying 86-87

Pyrazinamide: in tuberculosis, dosages 190-191

Q

Q fever: extrapulmonary manifestations 177

R

Radiation: long-term effects 161

Radiography
  chest
    in cough differential diagnosis 239
    in pulmonary embolism 250
    in liver cell adenoma 111-112
    in liver hyperplasia, focal nodular 114-115

Rai classification: of lymphocytic leukemia 148

Raynaud's phenomenon underlying conditions associated with 265

Regional enteritis
  differential diagnosis 91

Regurgitation
  aortic, causes 6
  mitral, causes 5-6
  tricuspid, causes 7

Reiter's syndrome
  clinical features suggesting 271
Renal disorders
  differential diagnosis
    acute glomerulonephritis
      214
    acute deterioration of renal
      function 208
  acute renal failure
    differential diagnosis of
      causative parenchymal
      renal diseases causing
      acute renal failure 208
  acute tubular injury
    differentiation of
      dehydration 213
  dialysis
    complications 229
  edema, generalized
    conditions leading to 223
  hematuria
    causes 230
  differential diagnosis
    nephrogenic diabetes
      insipidus 217
    nephrolithiasis 220
    nephrotic syndrome 214
  pulmonary syndromes 259
  renal complications of
    neoplasms 222
  transplants
    differential diagnosis of
      fever and pulmonary
      infiltrates in renal
      transplants 260
  tubulointerstitial disease of
    the kidney: differential
    diagnosis 279
  uremia
    clinical spectrum of
      abnormalities 224
Respiratory
  acidosis (See Acidosis,
    respiratory)
  alkalosis (See Alkalosis,
    respiratory)

disorders
  in mastocytosis 294
  predisposing to chronic cor
    pulmonale 28
  distress syndrome, adult,
    disorders associated
    with 251
  failure, differential
    diagnosis 245
Rheumatic fever
  diagnosis guidelines for initial
    attack 5
Rheumatoid arthritis
  revised classification
    criteria 270
  pulmonary manifestations 258
Rheumatoid factor:
  positive blood test for,
    differential diagnosis 275
Rheumatology: clinical 265-282
Rickets: classification 68-69
Rifampin: in tuberculosis,
  dosages 190-191
Roentgenography (See
  Radiography)
RTA (See Acidosis, rental tubular)

S

Salt
  bile, in malabsorption
    syndrome 88-89
  metabolism and
    corticosteroids 77-78
Sarcoid arthropathy 256
Sarcoidosis
  diagnostic features 274
Scleroderma (progressive
  systemic sclerosis)
    diagnostic criteria 267
Sedatives: in hepatic
  encephalopathy 108
Sella: empty sella syndrome,
  features associated with 46
Septal defect:
  atrial classification 7

Serostit 264
Shock
    cardiogenic 110
    causes 37
    initiating mechanisms 37
    toxic shock syndrome 187
SIADH 47-48
Sideroblastic anemia 133
Skin
    cancer 295-296
    disturbances in uremia 224
    lesions
        in cancer, internal 295-296
        in Reiter's syndrome 271
    manifestations
        of mastocytosis 294
        tumors in internal cancer
            295
Small intestine
    duodenal ulcer - refractory
        differential diagnosis 85
Sodium chloride 198
Sounds, second
    expiratory splitting, causes 2
    single sound, causes of 3
Spine: thoracic, diseases of 256
Spleen
    splenomegaly
        differential diagnosis 151
Spondylitis: ankylosing, diagnostic
    criteria 266
Stevens-Johnson syndrome
    diagnostic criteria 266
Stomach
    delayed gastric emptying 86
    hypergastrinemia
        conditions associated
            with 84
        Zollinger-Ellison syndrome
            (ZES) 84
Stones
    calcium
        formation 71
        in nephrolithiasis 220
    gallstone (See Gallstone)
    uric acid 220

Streptomycin: in tuberculosis,
    dosages 190
Stress: in hypertension 19
Sudden death
    nontraumatic 14
Surgery
    cardiovascular risk 31
Sweat gland disturbances 293
Syncope
    causes 21
Synovial fluid characteristics 280
Systemic lupus erythematosus
    diagnostic criteria 264

T

Tachyarrhythmia 21
Tamponade: common etiologies
    27
Target cells 143
TBG: altered concentration 51
T-cell deficiency syndrome 242
T₄: decreased peripheral
    conversion 53
Thioacetazone: in tuberculosis,
    dosages 190
Thrombocytes
    differential diagnosis
        thrombocytopenia 153
        thrombocytosis 147
        thrombotic thrombocytic
            purpura: diagnostic
                criteria 150
Thromboembolism
    risk factors 29
Thrombolism
    thrombolytic therapy
        Contraindications 39
Thrombotic thrombocytopenic
    purpura
        diagnostic criteria 150
Thyroid
    hyperthyroidism
        causes 49
        clinical features 49
    hypothyroidism
        clinical features 50

decreased conversion of T3 to T4 53
hypthyroidism
causes 50
TBG
altered concentrations 51
thyroid tumor
histological classification (WHO) 52
Thyroxine 53-54
TNM nomenclature: in lung cancer 157
Toxic shock syndrome 187
Toxicity
of chemotherapy, classification 160-161
Toxins
in ARDS 251
nephrotoxins, major 212
in renal tubulointerstitial disease 216-217
Tranquilizers: in hpeatic encephalopathy 108
Transplantation: renal, fever and pulmonary infiltrates in 260
Tricuspid regurgitation: causes 7
Triiodothyronine 53-54
TSH 49
T_3: decreased peripheral conversion 53
Tuberculosis
classification 173
drugs in, regimens 190
Tumor(s)
in FUO etiology 172
germ cell 256
hypercalcemia in 66
lung (See Lung tumors)
mesenchymal 256
multiple endocrine neoplasia syndrome 168
paraneoplastic 177
in renal tubulointerstitial disease 216
skin, in internal cancer 295
thyroid 52-53

U

Ulcer
in colitis (See Colitis, ulcerative)
duodenal, refractory, differential diagnosis 85
Uremia
anemia of 132
clinical spectrum of abnormalities in 224-225
Urethritis: in Reiter's syndrome 271
Uric acid 219
stones 220
Urinary tract
urinary tract obstruction differential diagnosis 210
tuberculosis: clinical features 173

V

Valve: pulmonary, insufficiency 29
Vascoconstrictor mechanisms 21-22
Vascular system
superior vena cava syndrome 163
Vasculitic syndromes
classification 277
Vasculitides: classification 227
Vena cava syndrome: superior 162
Ventilation: mechanical, with drawal from, guidelines 246
Ventricle
left, disease 13
right, hypertrophy 13
Vessels
(See also Cardiovascular)
in cancer, internal 295
disorders
in cancer, internal 295
of kidney, diseases 208
occlusion in Raynaud's phenomenon 265
risk in patients considered for surgery 31

Virus
  cytomegalovirus
    mononucleosis,
      features 179
  meningitis due to 284
Vitamin
  B$_{12}$ deficiency 133
  D metabolism abnormalities in
    hypophosphatemia 75

W

Water
  loss 203
  metabolism and
    corticosteroids 77-78
Weakness
  causes 21
White cells 280
Wilson's disease: diagnosis 117
Withdrawal: from mechanical
  ventilation, guidelines 246

X

X-ray (See Radiography)

Z

Zinc deficiency
  clinical features 91
Zollinger-Ellison syndrome:
  diagnosis 84